HEALING

Beyond Pills & Potions

HEALING

Beyond Pills & Potions

CORE PRINCIPLES FOR HEALERS & HELPERS

STEVE BIERMAN M.D.

"Man has received from nature both the destroyer of health and the preserver of health...; what the first strives to shatter and destroy, the innate physician repairs."

—Paracelsus

"To deprecate the higher emergent properties on the basis of their initial elemental building blocks is to further the error of materialistic thinking."

—Roger Sperry

"If he, Akbar, stepped outside the circle, could he live without its comforting circularity, in the terrifying strangeness of a new thought?"

—Salman Rushdie

The information given in this book should not be treated as a substitute for professional medical advice for any specific illness or condition. Always consult a medical practitioner for proper care and treatment. Any use of information in this book is at the reader's discretion and risk. Neither the author nor the publisher can be held responsible for any loss, claim or damage arising out of the use, or misuse, of the suggestions made, the failure to take medical advice or for any material in third-party websites.

Published in the United States of America by Gyro Press International, California.

Includes bibliographical references and index. Hardcover ISBN: 978-0-578-64370-0

Audiobook available at: **www.healingbeyondpills.com**

TABLE OF CONTENTS

Part III—*Artful Applications and Exquisite Outcomes*

"Discovery commences with the awareness of anomaly, i.e., with the recognition that nature has somehow violated the paradigm-induced expectations that govern normal science."

—Thomas Kuhn, *The Structure of Scientific Revolutions*

INTRODUCTION

I KNEW SOMETHING WAS WRONG with Western medicine at the end of my Family Practice residency. I hefted my patient Carol's three-inch-thick chart, filled with notes on her serial ailments and treatments over the last three years, and wondered: "Is this it? Is this what I'm going to be doing for the rest of my life—treating an endless stream of illnesses, one after the next, after the next, all the way to the grave?" It dawned on me in that moment that, while I was compassionately treating Carol's illnesses, I was doing little to restore her health—at least, in any lasting way. So, I retreated to the Emergency Department (ED), where I practiced as a board-certified physician for nearly 20 years.

It was spectacular. Nowhere else are the benefits of modern medicine more salient and sure. I felt purposeful and right. In those days, I would challenge any and all detractors of Western medicine by saying: "Why don't you follow me one Saturday night, just once…and then tell me what other kind of medicine you think would have been better for those sick and injured people."

But deep down I still knew something wasn't right. As magnificent as Western medicine is for treating emergencies and stabilizing extreme conditions, it did little or nothing to address what I was beginning to suspect were the deeper causes of many illnesses. Somewhere along the way, I had started asking my patients the most important question in medicine (that is, after the diagnosis has been secured)—namely, "Why today?" Why, when the world is bathed in bacteria, did you get pneumonia today? Why, when your cardiac lesion has been accumulating for years, did you have a heart attack today? You might have come down with appendicitis a week ago or a week from now—why today?

To my surprise, virtually every patient I asked had a plausible reason: "My mother-in-law just moved in with us." "I need to get out of this job, no matter what." "I just learned I was conned, and now I'm broke." Psychological reasons for physical maladies kept cropping up, again and again. And yet, my beloved science gave no ground to mental causes. Nothing in my training even allowed for the possibility. And if mental causes were excluded, what possible part could noetic (meaning: of or pertaining to the mind) factors play in a cure?

At the time, of course, I had no idea these nagging questions would lead me to hypnosis and compel me to untangle the tragic misconception that had relegated that world to "the fringe." Nor could I have realized, then, that finally understanding hypnosis would allow me to unlock the secrets of placebo and nocebo, and more broadly, to understand the impact of ideas on health and healing.

Nevertheless, along the way I had become sensitized to the influence all caregivers possess, to the impact of our words and deeds—sometimes for better and sometimes for worse. I learned that subtle refinements in our communications—and in our thoughts about causes and cures—could be integrated into our daily practice to improve actual outcomes and convey a sense of hope and alliance to patients. I also discovered, to my amazement, that those very same refinements could also be used to uproot the deep causes of many diseases and bring about lasting cures.

Exciting stuff for any healer. But during my early days in the Emergency Department, all of that lay ahead.

HEALING: BEYOND PILLS & POTIONS

Firewalking

Around the same time I began asking patients "Why today?" I took a surf trip to Bali. There one evening, I witnessed an entranced village elder dance over blazing hot coals for half-an-hour, without suffering so much as a blister. I was astounded. Not only did the fire dancer defy the "expectations that govern normal science," he also defied my own direct experience. As it happened, every July 5th in southern California, people would come screaming into the Emergency Department with second- and third-degree burns on their feet. Why? Because the previous day (4th July), when the celebratory beach barbeques were over, the revelers would bury their embers in the sand. The following morning, unsuspecting beachgoers would trample the coals and suffer the painful consequences. At the time, I could make no more sense of firewalking than I could of the possibility of psychological causes of illness. Both seemed somehow related to "the power of the mind." But what did that mean? So, I consigned firewalking to the category of "religious mysteries" and moved on.

That is until Tony Robbins started coaxing "regular people" over the coals. So much for my "religious mysteries" explanation. Naturally, when Robbins brought his fire pit seminar to San Diego, I went to watch. But instead, I walked. Firewalked. I knew I couldn't explain it, the firewalking, but now there was another equally perplexing question posed by the event. How did Tony Robbins manage to talk over 300 seemingly sensible individuals, including myself, into taking off their shoes and socks and parading over 10 meters of red-hot coals? During the two hours leading up to the walk, all he did was tell a tale or two. Or, so it seemed.

It turns out, Mr. Robbins was using a modeling technique known as Neuro-Linguistic Programming (NLP), which was the brainchild of Richard Bandler and John Grinder. Bandler and Grinder had managed to distill and methodize the bewildering techniques of the most eminent hypnotherapist of the day—Milton Erickson, M.D. For all my studies in Family Practice and Emergency Medicine, this was a world I knew nothing about. Quickly, I read *Uncommon Therapy* and realized that Erickson (who died in 1980) had singlehandedly figured out how to cure psychological maladies like no one else in the history of psychiatry or psychoanalysis. His methods were unconventional and ingenious. And Bandler and Grinder had dissected out the essential elements and were out there teaching.

So, in 1985, I flew to Philadelphia to study with John Grinder. It was the most brilliant and transformative seminar of my life. Those three days began a decade-long obsession with Erickson, NLP and hypnosis. I read everything I could; studied, practiced and eventually became Board Certified in Medical Hypnosis and credentialed in NLP. I applied the methods I was learning to virtually every situation I encountered in the ED and in the private Medical Hypnosis practice I established. At first, I "hypnotized" patients to help relieve their pain and anxiety—something I was constantly witnessing in the ED. And it worked. Kids drifted off "to Disneyland," and let me suture their lacerations without having to restrain them. Adults settled into a quiet, comfortable repose, without requiring much in the way of analgesia or anesthesia. Soon I was performing all kinds of potentially painful procedures without provoking so much as a whimper. As my confidence grew, I started doing what ED doctors do—winging it. I offered suggestions for more than just comfort and relief. I suggested that bleeding stop, joints relocate after dislocation, heart rhythms normalize. Much to my amazement, these suggestions also worked—sometimes with and, even more surprisingly, sometimes without a formal trance induction. It wasn't long before I was publishing extraordinary case reports in major medical journals and national television networks were sending crews to film me. It was a marvelous time. I was witnessing miracles, even while learning how to bring them about. Things were rolling.

Non-surgical Cure

Then, I got sick. As the CT scan confirmed, an intervertebral disc between C4 and C5 in my neck had ruptured. The pain was excruciating, and the arm that was innervated by the compressed nerve was becoming impossibly weak. Unfortunately, I hadn't yet learned how to turn the powers of hypnosis on myself. So, instead, I turned to my trusted medical colleagues. "Here is what we'll do," they explained, confidently. "First, we'll cut into your neck from the front—being careful not to nick the carotid arteries, of course." They could have stopped there, but they didn't. "Then, we'll spread open the space with traction and remove the faulty disc." At that point, I'm pretty sure my decision was made. "Then, we'll hammer in a piece of your hip bone—"

Enough!

The quest for a non-surgical cure was on. I started reading, desperately, while taking pills to ease the pain. I read about homeopathy, osteopathy, chiropractic, naturopathy and much more. I tried several of these worthy disciplines—but to no avail. Finally, after finishing Michael Harner's *The Way of the Shaman* and several other scholarly texts on shamanic healing, I convinced a physician friend of mine to accompany me on a trip to Ecuador.

After a few missteps, we found a guide, Jose, who claimed to be a "Brujo-in-training" (a Brujo is a shaman). With him, we took a dirt road out of the small town of Macas to its terminus. Then, the three of us traipsed through boot-sucking mud, inched over furious rivers on slippery log bridges and slogged deep into the jungle. Hours later, we reached the Brujo's encampment, where 13 puzzled patients asked: "What took you so long? We've been waiting two hours." They explained that two hours prior to our arrival, the Brujo had a vision of two white men coming toward them. "We shall wait," he declared. And so, they did.

That night, after taking the medicine—Ayahuasca, the jungle vision vine— the Brujo treated all 13 patients. Many of them described themselves as cured on the spot. The next night, the Brujo again took Ayahuasca. As the visions commenced, he examined me by peering through a crystal as he passed it over my body, up and down. When he came to the left side of my neck, at the level of the ruptured disc, he paused. Mind you, I had simply asked for an examination, telling him nothing of my ailment. Then, he drew a deep breath and blew. It felt like an Arctic wind whose full force had somehow focused on my neck. I remember shivering. Again, the Brujo blew. And again, the freeze. Then, he held the crystal over my neck and declared: "Curado!" And cured I was. Within days I no longer needed the pills I had been taking—the pain was gone. Soon, the strength in my arm returned, and shortly thereafter I was able to recommence all my sports and work activities.

* * *

The anomalies—things conventional science just could not explain—were stacking up. I had already consigned firewalking to the cabinet of mysteries. I had no explanation for the consistently plausible "Why today?" answers my patients were offering. I had the accumulating wonders of NLP and hypnosis I was, literally, witnessing every day at work. And now, I had this jungle ritual, which entailed nothing more than me holding still while an inebriated tribal elder huffed and puffed. How could his actions have possibly restored what was clearly a mechanical injury deep in my spinal column? I was hearing faint echoes from Andrew Weil's thought-provoking *Health and Healing:* "I find allopathic medicine glaringly deficient in theory and philosophy of any sort."

Of course, my surgical colleagues shrugged it off. "Placebo effect," they declared as if to say…bogus! "It will be back."

"Nice," I thought. First, the meaningless dismissal of a glaring fact (i.e., I was back at work, despite not having succumbed to surgery); and then, the curse ("it will be back"). Sadly, I began to hear this pattern repeated frequently by my colleagues—not all of them, but many—most of whom I knew to be earnest and compassionate caregivers. It was as if they had been taught this quick thrust and facile parry as a defense against all things inexplicable.

Chinese Energy Healing

Not long after these events, curiosity led me to study with Sifu Share K. Lew, a Taoist priest and Nui-Gung Grandmaster. A kind and encyclopedic teacher, Sifu was also a powerful healer who explained that his cures resulted from changing body-energetics—removing blocks and restoring the flow of *chi* energy. Coming from southern California, I was especially dubious of all things "energy." I understood the energy of physics; it was quantifiable and subject to the Laws of Nature. But I recoiled at the ill-defined "energy" of alternative medicine: as in, "Her energy isn't balanced" or "This manipulation will shift your energy." Nevertheless, I could feel the *chi* Sifu was pushing out of his hands, and I had direct sensory experiences with the energies he called "yin" and "yang."

Moreover, I witnessed many of his cures. For example, I saw and traced with X-rays, Sifu's healing of a young man with a non-union of the navicular bone. The orthopedist had urged a surgical repair and yet, despite having persisted for more than two years, Sifu's methods somehow knitted the fragments together within a matter of weeks. I also witnessed a woman in her 30's, who had been branded "a nutcase" after years of cyclic abdominal pain, who was cured in two sessions by Sifu's ministrations. And there were dozens more. As to his "energy," I once watched him project his chi across a room, at a skeptical patient's back, while she sat facing away from him on the floor. Within minutes, she grew hotter and hotter, her face redder and sweatier, until at length she could take no more: "Okay, okay!" she protested. "I'm a believer."

And so was I.

Until I read an account by Dr. James Esdaile (written in 1846), wherein he induced the exact same changes in a "hypnotic subject" through the subtle transmission from his fingertips of so-called Mesmeric fluid.

***

At this point, my mind was a whirl of confusion—anomalies everywhere. There were only three things I could be sure of. First, I wasn't about to give up conventional allopathic medicine. I had seen what it could do, and it was a lifesaver. Second, I knew from direct experience that hypnosis, shamanic healing and Chinese energy healing worked. I had no idea how they worked or what, if anything, might be their common thread, but I wasn't about to dismiss these modalities (or other complementary disciplines) by pretending they were bogus. Third, I had seen enough in my years since medical school to know our science was incomplete. The Bard was right: "There are more things in heaven and Earth...than are dreamt of in your philosophy." And those "things" included the marvels I was witnessing in the ED and my private office every day: patients responding not only with relief from pain and anxiety but also with phenomenal physical changes, such as the cessation of bleeding, the normalization of aberrant heart rhythms, bloodless surgeries, relaxation of airways and the disappearance of tumors.

In the face of such stupendous anomalies, the peremptory dismissals and negative suggestions of my colleagues seemed feckless and small. Mental matters had been roundly excluded from my medical education, yet kept evincing themselves as powerful elements in the interplay of causes and cures. Without somehow factoring in the agency of Mind, modern medicine could hope for nothing better than what I had come to recognize as the blunt beginnings and endless endings of serial ailments and infirmities.

The Exquisite Art of Caregiving

Healing: Beyond Pills and Potions is the result of my decades-long effort to resolve this confusion—not by discarding Western medicine, but by expanding it. The end result is a wider command of the healing arts and a deeper sense of personal fulfillment in caregiving.

We begin our journey by learning that the state of helplessness and dependency, common to many if not most sick patients, triggers a primordial survival reflex. This reflex scans for The One least uncertain, and vests that one with what I will call "Authority." Not the authority of a boss or police officer, but rather, the Authority of a newborn's parent—the provider and protector of life itself. As such, ideas flow unimpeded from Authority to subject, from caregiver to patient. Mind Matters.

We then learn how Authority features in the rituals of all healers, from the ancients of prehistory to the Asclepians of Greece to the placebo-controlled trials of modern medicine. And we discover, therein, the first of many secrets—the implicit structure behind the Placebo Effect, and its ability to help or harm.

And so, we consider first how to avoid harm. We learn what constitutes a negative suggestion and how to avoid inadvertently hurling curses. We examine the dangers of the common Fallacies of Extrapolation and Prophecy. And we contemplate Therapeutic Restraint, in the context of reverence for the Wisdom of the Body and charitable forgiveness for our own inevitable mistakes.

Then, we turn to helping, to using our words and deeds to produce positive outcomes. This is where we begin to witness the wondrous exercise of "mind over matter"—bloodless surgeries, shrinking tumors, "chronic" illnesses (both physical and mental) interrupted and dispelled. It is also where the real work begins. Where new communication habits are formed and fashioned. But it is joyful work, rich in its rewards. For here we learn how to deliver information honestly, in a manner that leaves our patients hopeful and impelled toward health.

Soon, however, the unspoken underpinnings of conventional medicine begin to constrain us, and we are forced to reckon with reductionism's implied notion of causality, a causality that excludes all things psychological. It is a worthy exercise, though; for at its conclusion we are left with a humanistic causal model—one that includes the truncated sequences of our science, even as it expands to allow for both mental and physical causes and cures. And once again, a secret is revealed—this time the source of Ockham's razor, the diagnostic principle that guides most conventional allopathic practitioners.

The reach of our new model is pervasive, touching literally every aspect of caregiving: from taking a patient's history, to formulating a diagnosis and treatment plan, to delivering a deep and lasting cure. This is a transformative undertaking–one that drives us to continually improve our communications and refine our thinking, so that our patients may reap the full benefits we now realize are possible. No longer must they suffer painful procedures or bloody surgeries. No longer must they linger under the curse of chronicity, without hope and alliance.

Often our goals can be achieved using simple refinements in our basic gestural and linguistic toolbox. But not always. There are times when circumstances are so dire or causes so deep that more powerful tools and more protracted encounters are necessary. Enter, hypnosis. But not the hypnosis you might think. Not the hypnosis that, for centuries, has been conflated with trance. Instead, we discover that what drives hypnotic responses are certain simple behavioral patterns we can establish with our patients. These patterns drive our suggestions to actualization. While trance can be a response to certain sets of suggestions, health and healing can be responses to other sets of suggestions. Trance, in other words, is an effect. Hypnosis is the cause. Once this is understood and clarified, a universe of salutary outcomes blooms before us.

What emerges from these various considerations is what I call the Exquisite Art of Caregiving—using words and deeds to help and heal. No matter whether you are a well-meaning relative assisting an ailing loved one, a chiropractor or surgeon, midwife or naturopath, Emergency Physician or acupuncturist—I am confident the skills and teachings in this book will enrich your practice and enhance your love of caregiving.

PART I

Elements of the Art

We begin by asking, "Isn't it enough to be a compassionate caregiver?" After all, the germs, cells and molecules that cause illness are not thinking things. They are mindless materials subject to the laws of science. Why should it matter what we say or do, so long as we offer the proper treatment compassionately?

It is a fair question. But as we are about to learn, there is more to health and healing than material science. Mind Matters. The ideas presented by caregivers can both harm and heal. And so, we begin our exploration of the Exquisite Art of Caregiving by refining our communication skills—learning what to say and how best to say it—and by acquiring the necessary wisdom to achieve the outcomes our patients desire and deserve.

"The profession of medicine is like that of music.
You never stop learning and improving your technique."

—Manuel Cordova-Rios, *Rio Tigre and Beyond*

Chapter 1:
COMPASSION IS NOT ENOUGH

A SIMPLE QUESTION. Which would you prefer? A compassionate doctor who says, "Don't worry, although 90% of patients die from your condition, no matter how dreadful the struggle, I will be with you and care for you to the very end."

Or, a dispassionate doctor who says, "Listen, 10% of people—very much like yourself—survive this diagnosis. [Same statistical information, but with an implied survival suggestion.] And, there is a new treatment that may even improve those odds. [Knowledge, pure and simple.] I suggest we go down this new path together and that…you become a survivor. [Creating a sense of alliance while, again, embedding a strong survival suggestion.]"

In this case, the answer is obvious. Anyone wishing to survive will choose the dispassionate doctor with knowledge and wisdom.

Compassion is not enough. Patients do not need their professional caregivers to hold their hands and cry with them. They need their caregivers to use every bit of information and every modicum of skill they possess to minimize suffering and maximize health. The time for shared tears may come, but most often abundant opportunities to effect positive change precede those moments. Effective caregivers—driven by compassion—practice the Exquisite Art of Caregiving. As we shall see, this precious art affects not only attitudes but also outcomes.

Compassion from a caregiver, in the absence of knowledge and wisdom, can do real harm. Sometimes that harm is psychological. Sometimes it is physical. Often, it is both. Here are some examples:

"Psychological" Pain

The ambulance arrives with an 80-year-old woman, Rose, complaining of sudden excruciating pain in her right lower extremity. Her gray hair is piled high and messy with sweat. Her gentle features contorted in agony. She moans and writhes inconsolably.

On examination, her heartbeat is irregular. Her right lower extremity is pale and pulseless from groin to foot. It is a simple diagnosis: a blood clot has dislodged from her fibrillating heart and completely obstructed the large artery to the leg. If the clot is not removed soon, she will lose her leg and possibly her life.

Morphine offers scant relief. We give more. And more.

The surgeon is called. He is exceptional. I've known John since our training days. Good hands, good heart. He has chosen to live close to the hospital so he can respond quickly to his patients' needs.

Four agonizing minutes till he arrives.

I have called the operating room in advance. They refuse to open a new suite, to call in another team. The hip fracture they are currently operating on will be done in 30–45 minutes. "You'll just have to wait."

The patient's screams intensify.

John, the surgeon, arrives, receives my report and examines the patient. Irate at the delay, he lifts the bedside phone. Rose hears every word he

HEALING: BEYOND PILLS & POTIONS

bellows: "Dammit, if I can't get this patient into surgery within 15 minutes, she will lose her leg!" He slams the phone down and storms off.

The patient twists in agony. Each second an eternity....

John is the most compassionate surgeon I know. He studied long and hard to become a superlative operator. Like many, he assumed his innate compassion would inform his communications sufficiently. It did not. The psychological pain Rose suffered after that horrifying phone call could easily have been avoided with a few well-chosen words. After slamming the phone down, for example, John could have turned and said softly:

"Sometimes I have to scream to get their attention. [Synchronizing his breathing with the patient—as a subtle way to initiate Rapport.] Rest assured, Rose, we will save your leg. Relief is near. [Placing his hand gently on her shoulder—thereby diverting a portion of her attention from the leg.] Very near. I'm with you...."

Creating *Rapport*, suggesting relief, while offering hope and alliance—these are all aspects of the Exquisite Art of Caregiving: aspects I will elaborate on extensively in the coming chapters. They distinguish the artist from the artisan, the elegant cure from the inadvertent curse.

Rose's leg was ultimately saved, though dreams of lost limbs haunted her.

***

Here is another example, this one more common though perhaps less obvious:

"Physical" Pain

The child is scared. He knows he is about to get a shot.

Out of compassion—not wishing to startle the boy or lose trust— the nurse cautions, "a little bee sting" or "a little prick," as she brings the needle near.

The boy braces himself, teeth clenched. Then, the pain, the tears.

The nurse feels justified. At least she warned him.

Compassion alone can cause kids to cry and adults to wince.

Thousands of clinicians do this every day. They believe shots must hurt. Therefore, warning someone of the impending pain is better than surprising them. These same compassionate individuals have no idea they are, in fact, offering a self-fulfilling prophecy. The pain they witness is the inevitable outcome of their own negative suggestions, not of the needle.

I have given more than 1,100 injections painlessly, and I can assert with absolute certainty: there is nothing inevitable about an injection being painful. Of course, a patient on high alert and in "feeling-mode" (i.e., mentally searching for "a bee sting") will experience a shot as painful. However, the wise application of two simple principles (first, focus attention; and second, direct that attention away from feelings) will invariably render injections painless.

For example, instead of the compassionate "bee sting" warning:

1. "Now listen closely, this is important."

(Something important is about to be said...what? Confusion, even momentary, focuses attention.)

2. "In a second or two, you'll hear a peculiar crunch...JUST listen."

("Just" means "and nothing else." If they JUST listen, they do not feel.)

As they listen intently, you inject—painlessly.

    Or,

1. "Now I need you to look over there at that orange circle-square...really look...and tell me if it moves up or down."

(There is no such thing as a "circle-square," so it's confusing: Attention focuses as the patient tries to locate and make sense of it. You sound earnest, so there must be something out there.)

2. "It's important, so JUST look."

(If they JUST look, again, they do not feel.)

Again, you inject—painlessly.

I've taught this simple technique to hundreds of caregivers. Can you imagine their surprise upon discovering how easy it is to deliver painless injections? And how gratifying? A few well-chosen words.

* * *

Another illustration:

Anxiety and Bleeding

Most nights around 7pm, a patient arrives in the Emergency Department with pulsatile bleeding from a finger laceration. The story goes as follows:

The patient was washing/drying a glass after dinner and it broke, cutting the finger and slicing through a small digital artery. Direct pressure has been applied, often for an hour or more, but to no avail. Hence, the ED visit.

As a young physician, I would often introduce myself to such a patient and say: "I'm sorry I can't get to your wound quite yet. As you can probably see, we have some pressing emergencies right now. However, I see you've lost a lot of blood, so I've asked the technician to apply a pressure dressing. Just know, as soon as I can return, I'll be back and take care of you." I would say this in full earnest and with real compassion.

Not bad, really. Compassionate. But those words do nothing to stop bleeding and little to allay anxiety.

Later in my career I learned to say, "You must have been a bit worried, weren't you, over that bleeding?" (Thus, placing their fear in the past.)

"And yet now, I'm going to ask you to do something, and I'm sure you'll think I'm kidding, but I'm not. I really do mean it. And you might even want to laugh a little…

"But [synching my breathing to theirs, exuding earnest] I need you to… stop your bleeding…now." (My tone certain, our eyes locked, my head gently nodding.)

Odd as it may sound, and I know it does sound odd at first, virtually all such patients respond as follows: First, they chuckle timidly (as predicted); then, perceiving my earnest, they hush; and finally, they watch in amazement as the bleeding, beat-by-beat, first slows and then, seconds later, stops.

"That's right," I affirm confidently. Then, turning to the technician, "Please dress the wound. I'll be back shortly to close it properly."

Again, compassion is not enough—not when a few well-chosen words can extinguish anxiety and halt bleeding.

***

Here is one final example. It teaches how one misplaced word, **"you,"** can transform a well-intended communication into a dreadful curse.

To Curse or Cure

On the other side of the curtain, I hear a physician giving informed consent to his patient, regarding an antihypertensive (blood pressure) medicine. Informed consent, which is required unless expressly waived by the patient, is the explanation in simple terms of all potential risks and benefits.

"So I believe all your symptoms are the result of high blood pressure. The good news is we can treat that with a medicine called Atenolol™.

HEALING: BEYOND PILLS & POTIONS

Now, like all medicines, Atenolol has both risks and benefits, which I am obliged to explain to you."

"Okay, Doctor, if you must."

"The benefits are easy—it can lower your blood pressure and make you feel a whole lot better. We've known each other for a long time, Todd, and I sure would like you to feel better."

"Me too, Doc."

*"The risks…well, the risks of Atenolol are…it could cause **you** to faint or feel queasy; it could cause **you** to become impotent, or **your** heart to miss beats—sometimes a lot of beats—even to the point of passing out; or, in the worst case, it could kill **you**—"*

"Kill me? Doctor, I'm—"

"But it's not gonna kill you, Todd, I just mean it could. For goodness sake, an aspirin can kill you if you're allergic or have an ulcer…"

It's important to know that a caregiver's words can affect clinical outcomes. A positive suggestion, implied or expressed, can produce a positive outcome—this is the Placebo Effect. Whereas, a negative suggestion can produce a negative outcome—the so-called Nocebo Effect. Virtually every placebo-controlled clinical trial ever conducted has contained placebo/nocebo responders. I will have much more to say about this in the next chapter. For now, bear in mind, the caregiver's words cut both ways.

When a doctor says of a proposed treatment "it could kill **you**," he or she is unintentionally directing a negative suggestion at the patient. The doctor could have said, with equal ease and accuracy:

*"Many patients, like **you**, experience a pleasant and uneventful lowering of blood pressure with Atenolol. However, there are **some patients** who experience untoward side effects [listing them].*

*Although very rare, **some people** could even die. Please call me tomorrow and let me know how well **you** are doing."*

"You" versus "some patients/some people." One word ("you") directs the curse; the other words ("some patients/some people") deflect it. A powerful distinction and, as we will learn, an important one in the Exquisite Art of Caregiving.

Summing Up

Without compassion there would be no caregivers. But compassion alone is not enough; in its raw form, it can mislead and misdirect. As I said earlier, patients do not need their professional caregivers to simply hold their hands and cry with them. Compassionate friends and family can do that. **For the professional caregiver, compassion should fuel the endless quest for knowledge and wisdom.**

The following chapters explore what years of compassion-driven practice, reading, failing and succeeding have taught me. In it, you'll discover there is a right way to provide information to patients: a method for delivering diagnoses, treatment plans and informed consent that invariably creates a sense of hope and alliance while effecting positive outcomes. You'll learn how to instill curative suggestions that can and often do work wonders, to perform painless procedures, to allay anxieties and to influence surgical outcomes. Along the way, we'll plumb the causes of symptom formation and probe the mysteries of hypnosis, and I will offer hints at how to effect positive outcomes with a few well-chosen words and well-timed gestures. I will share with you my successes—e.g., biopsy-proven tumors cured, autoimmune diseases reversed, psychiatric illnesses allayed, bloodless surgeries performed, fatal arrhythmias normalized, dislocated joints reduced. And I will examine my failures and their consistent causes.

There is much to master, so let's begin.

"As a man imagines himself, so shall he be."

—Paracelsus, *Paracelsus: Selected Writings*

Chapter 2:
Mind Matters

IF IDEAS CAN AFFECT PHYSICAL HEALTH, then our words and actions as caregivers are much more important than we may realize.

IF a patient's ideas can cause illness, then as caregivers we must learn to ask a whole new range of questions from those currently required in the "history of the present illness."

IF ideas can cure, then caregivers must learn how and when to offer salutary suggestions most effectively.

Of course, none of these "If's" are addressed in traditional caregiver training. Why? Because reductionist science and simplistic causal notions ignore the emergent properties of the whole person (e.g., volition, imagination, thought), reducing health and healing to the mindless materiality of cells and molecules. If a microbe is deemed the first and final cause of a patient's illness, then killing that microbe is all that matters. There is no mystery in the history. No secret in the send-off—in what you say regarding the treatment plan and prognosis. Prescribe the drug that kills the bug, and your job is done.

It was only at the end of my three-year Family Medicine residency that I began to doubt this reductionist model. I remember holding the ponderous chart of Carol, one of my favorite patients. A pleasant lady in her mid-50s, Carol loved seeing me and said so at every visit. Over the years, I had treated her for hypertension, strep throat, vaginosis, autoimmune disease and numerous other ailments. But no matter how effective the treatment, she always returned a month or two later with some new malady. After three years, I couldn't help but wonder: Is this really "healing," this extended exercise in repairs and replacements, in measurements and medications? And if so, how could I explain those patients who saw me only once or twice during the same period? Or those "tough old-timers" who never saw me or any physician and did just fine. Was Carol just cursed with "bad protoplasm?" Were those other people just gifted with "good genes?" Possibly.

However, another possibility began to fascinate me—namely, that a patient's unconscious ideas might act as potent contributory factors in the causal sequences leading to illness. The question was, how to bring those ideas to light? Eventually, I discovered that by asking patients one simple question I could often unearth the very ideas that seemed to be adversely affecting their health.

Let's begin our exploration of the noetic causes of illness with that very question, which now forms a key element in the Exquisite Art of Caregiving.

"If You Had to Guess… Why Today?"

It's a busy afternoon in the Emergency Department. I have to keep moving from room to room, patient to patient. No time to waste.

Greg is a 38-year-old married man complaining of left testicular pain. He denies sex outside of marriage or unusual exposures. He has no fever or chills; laboratory tests, including urinalysis and blood counts, are normal. His physical examination reveals a tender epididymis (the structure atop the testis), non-tender testicles, no discharge or lymphadenopathy. A urethral swab is sent for culture and antibiotic sensitivities.

Greg has epididymitis, etiology unknown. Possible causes are legion, ranging from mild trauma (which he denies) to vasculitis to infection. I treat him with antibiotic and anti-inflammatory medication and refer him for follow-up to the urologist. Bug–drug–done.

I have to move on. Others are waiting. Still, I can't resist asking: "Greg, I know you won't know the answer to this. But this condition could probably have occurred yesterday or the day before… or maybe even a week ago. Again, I know you don't know…but if you had to guess… why do you think you came down with this today?" (Remember this question and how I framed it.)

At this point, I had been working for over 10 years as an Emergency Physician. Experience had taught me that once the diagnosis is made, this is the single most important question one can ask a patient. Greg's answer was typical:

"Gee, I don't know, Doc," he mutters, pulling up his pants. "Haven't got a clue."

"I know you don't know…but if you had to guess?"

Silence. A familiar silence, and one I've learned to wait out.

"Doc?" Greg finally asks, buckling his belt: "Do you think this will prevent me from getting that vasectomy tomorrow? My wife is really insisting on it."

There it is. I just had to wait for it. The wish: I wish I could get out of the vasectomy. The fulfillment: retreat into illness.

"You can pretty much be certain no surgeon will operate in a possibly infected field," I say. "Most likely, the surgery will have to be postponed."

Is Greg's answer unusual? Are purposeful symptoms a rarity?

In my experience, the answer to the question, "Why today? Just guess," is quite often tendential. You have to ask the question correctly. You have to restrain yourself during the inevitable silence that follows. It takes practice and patience. But no single question will yield more precious insights into the possible psychological causes of your patients' illnesses than "Why today?

Just guess." I could give you hundreds of examples. Here are a few:

"Why today (Why now)?...Just guess."

Appendicitis patients: "Why today? Just guess."
—30-year-old female: "I don't know, but can they unblock my fallopian tubes while they are in there? We couldn't afford the procedure, but our insurance covers anything through the ED. And now, we really want to have a baby."

—Overworked medical intern: "I don't know, but I sure can use the rest."

Mouth sores (aphthous ulcers): "Why today? Just guess."
—42-year-old male: "No idea, Doc...say, will these prevent me from having my wisdom tooth removed tomorrow?"

Breast cancer: "Why today? Just guess."
—47-year-old female: Guilt—extramarital affair.

—36-year-old female: Guilt—abortion.

Autoimmune disease: "Why today? Just guess."
—39-year-old female, lupus: Guilt—family member suicide.

Vaginismus: "Why now? Just guess."
—44-year-old female: "I don't know, but I never want to be that vulnerable again."

Infection (meningococcemia): "Why today? Just guess."
—33-year-old physician, frustrated with hospital staffing, who one day earlier had said to himself: "I have to get outta this job, no matter what!"

Hand warts: "Why today? Just guess."
—Surgeon: "I wish I could retire and never have to operate again."

Heart attack: "Why today? Just guess."
—67-year-old male: "Mother-in-law showed up today for a five-month stay."

—Numerous other patients: Financial problems, romantic difficulties, moving.

Palpitations: "Why now? Just guess."

—63-year-old lawyer: "I don't know.… You don't think I'm trying to manufacture some physical reason to quit work, so that I don't seem like I'm intentionally betraying my partners, do you?"

As I said, many patients—provided you are hushed enough to wait for their answer—will come up with a "guess" that seems implicated in the etiology of their disease. Frequently, within that "guess" is a wish, like "I wish I could avoid this situation." Rarely, do patients allow such wishes to enter conscious thought; rather, their unhealthy wishes are suppressed into the realm most often referred to as the unconscious or subconscious. Even guilt, as we'll discuss in detail later, contains for many people the subconscious wish for punishment as a means of absolution.

Remember your own childhood? Wasn't there a time when some impending humiliation or challenge caused you to wish you could avoid going to school: a test, a performance, a bully? And then, shortly thereafter, didn't you discover with a peculiar sense of relief that your stomach ached, or your throat hurt, or you had a fever, dizziness, nausea…something? **The wish: I wish I didn't have to go. The fulfillment: retreat into illness.** Almost everyone raised in modern society has had this experience.

Of course, these considerations do not prove the notion that ideas can affect health. But, at the very least, they conjure the specter of plausibility. The proof will come soon enough, when we consider the Placebo Effect. But first, let's explore some other implications of our reasoning.

The Door Swings Both Ways

If an idea can make you sick, then another idea can make you well.

Think about it for a moment.… What happened when, as a child, your impending humiliation or challenge passed? Did the sore throat or tummy ache persist? No, at least, not for most of you. Instead, the wish to stay home (to retreat into illness) gave way to the wish to rejoin your friends (to return to health). Soon, you were well. One might wonder: Did the wish to retreat into illness simply abate and thereby allow the body's homeostatic systems to restore balance? Or, did the wish to get well itself somehow activate or potentiate the healing systems? Or, since these options are not mutually exclusive, did both occur?

This is no doubt an intriguing question for future noetic scientists. Meantime, there is plenty of evidence to suggest that salutary ideas can activate potent systems whose capacities to forestall illness and promote healing are both real and startling. Let's consider some of the evidence.

Forestalling Illness

Researchers at the University of California, San Diego have shown that in the weeks prior to major "Positive Life Events," mortality rates for affected groups fall. For example, among Chinese people the death rate falls by 35% in the two weeks leading up to Chinese New Year. Similarly, among Jewish people the mortality rate falls significantly in all three leading causes of death during the week before Passover. In both populations, these effects are statistically significant.

What is happening? How is it that an approaching holiday can push the pause button on death?

I think of it this way. These patients have a deep, unambivalent wish: "I wish to stay alive through this holiday season!" They are actuarially "scheduled" to die, but somehow their wish to live is pre-emptive. Survival mechanisms activate, enabling patients to "cheat death"—not forever, but long enough to make it through the holiday season with their families.

The door has swung the other way, this time toward survival.

Promoting Healing

Now let's look at a dramatic example of ideas influencing health and healing—presurgical hypnosis. This is a topic wherein I have perhaps more experience than most, having personally performed presurgical hypnosis for more than 40 years on scores and scores of patients. I will tell you now, there is nothing in the Exquisite Art that is more gratifying and astounding. And nothing easier. Here is my most recent case.

> Rick has an unfortunate diagnosis, rectal cancer. He has completed chemotherapy and radiation and is scheduled for surgery to remove his rectum and distal sigmoid colon. Recovery from this procedure can be protracted and painful. As with all presurgical hypnosis patients, to "build response potential," I declined to treat him in the days and weeks leading up to surgery.

> It is now the night before. His sense of helplessness and dependency is intense. Now is the time. Before the trance we agree on the three goals shared by all surgical patients: a "dry field" (i.e., no blood loss or, stated in positive terms, "keep your own blood"); delightfully surprising comfort; and really rapid wound healing. Rick adds two personal goals—normal post-operative bowel and sexual function.

> As do all patients in his predicament, Rick responds well to suggestions and experiences a light trance. I offer the agreed-upon salutary ideas in three ways—directly ("Keep your own blood"), indirectly ("You can forget to feel and *just know* what to move and not move…"), and metaphorically ("Imagine a **dry field**, vast and interminable…"). I also anticipate what experience has taught me will inevitably happen: "And as well-meaning people ask, 'How's your _pain_?' and 'What level is your _pain_?' and 'Would you like a _pain_ pill?' your unconscious will use the word PAIN as a trigger to, **Rick, feel even more comfortable.**"

He wakes with partial amnesia, feeling refreshed and alert. As we say good-bye, I end with: "Don't be opposed to pleasantly surprising yourself." He smiles wanly.

A week later, I receive his call. "You won't believe this, Doc. All I've taken since I woke from surgery is Tylenol. The surgeon couldn't believe it, so she gave me one dose of Toradol™; but I've declined all other meds."

"And was there any blood loss?" I ask.

"The surgeon told me it was minimal, almost none."

"And how about healing?"

"Well, I got out of the hospital a day early. The nurse who manages my stoma (a temporary ostomy) says she's never seen anything like it."

"Like what?" I ask.

"The healing. She says the stoma and my surgical wounds are healing faster than ever."

I remind Rick, as I've learned to remind all such patients: Remember, if your surgeon wants to remove your stitches in 14 days, be sure you schedule an appointment two days earlier. "Definitely", he says triumphantly.

Not only have ideas (i.e., suggestions) obviated pain, ideas have also prevented bleeding and accelerated healing. You may argue, "It's a series of one." It is not. I have had numerous astonished surgeons report bloodless surgeries to me on scores of patients, including those who have undergone the following procedures:

- total colectomy and hemicolectomy
- total shoulder replacement
- total knee replacement
- radical prostatectomy

- multiple abdominal and thoracic procedures
- hip replacements
- open heart surgery

...to name a few. Additionally, virtually every one of these patients experienced rapid wound healing, to the extent that their surgeons have remarked: "Gee, I'm glad you came in early, otherwise I might have had to dig these sutures out."

This is nothing new. In 1846, Dr. James Esdaile reported: "In surgery, the benefits of Mesmerism are not confined to the extinction of pain during an operation, but are of the greatest general and particular advantage in the after-treatment of surgical diseases." The astonished British surgeon goes on to detail scores of cases (including amputations) in which his highly dependent patients complied entirely with his implicit commands for comfort, relief and rapid wound healing.

Some of you may be thinking: *Cool stuff, indeed, but I don't know how to induce a hypnotic trance. So what use is all that to me?* Fair enough. Later, we will explore the nature of trance and the Hypnotic Method; thereafter, we will review a simple protocol for inducing bloodless surgeries and rapid wound healing. For now, it is sufficient to understand that hypnosis is merely a way of driving ideas to actualization. As such, presurgical hypnosis offers us compelling evidence that ideas can positively affect both psychological and physical responses. Mind Matters.

Next, let's turn to an even more compelling body of proof—placebo-controlled clinical trials.

Lessons from Placebo

For over 70 years, placebo-controlled trials have been the mainstay of medical science. Rigorously comparing a neutral substance or sham intervention to a new pill or procedure has enabled many of the advancements of conventional medicine that we currently treasure. At the same time, this abundant body of research has also shown us that placebo itself is capable of inducing therapeutic effects across a vast array of maladies. For example, placebo has been shown to lower blood sugar (18.7%), reduce the frequency of kidney stones (62%), lower high blood pressure (15–60%), improve arthritis and autoimmune syndromes (50%), better stroke outcomes (42.5%), effect coronary artery reperfusion at one-week post-infarction (41%), reduce the pain of diabetic neuropathic (51%), allay non-ulcer dyspepsia (25%), soothe chronic fatigue syndrome (37%) and ameliorate depression (55.6%)—to name a few Placebo Effects (and the percentage of patients responding). I should emphasize that these are not only psychological effects; in fact, they are primarily physical outcomes. (See: www.http://programinplacebostudies.org/publications/)

Yet, despite this long and consistent history, misconceptions about placebo abound. Generally, people assume a placebo works because patients believe it will work. They then reduce that belief to some "neurobiological substrate" (today, neurotransmitters; tomorrow, who knows) and bask in the comfort of a quasi-scientific explanation.

But, belief is not what powers placebo. If it were, then the roughly 25–35% of placebo-responders in the control groups (a rough average) must be those persons who believe most strongly. And the other 65–75% placebo non-responders must be those who believe less or not at all? There is no evidence to support this. Besides, believe in what? The belief has to be that the intervention (drug, procedure, etc.) will work as prescribed. But all participants in placebo-controlled clinical trials know they are in such a trial; therefore, they know that there is a 50/50 chance they are getting placebo and not the intervention. So, their belief is vitiated by doubt. Moreover, they know that there is uncertainty as to whether the intervention itself even works—hence, the trial. So, the belief of patients involved in placebo-controlled trials is at best partial, and certainly never absolute.

Yet, absolute belief does exist in some patients. What about the millions of people around the world who repose unalloyed faith in religious methods of treatment? According to the belief hypothesis, these patients should all be

HEALING: BEYOND PILLS & POTIONS

cured. Similarly, if belief were the sole desideratum, shouldn't every psychotic and every hypochondriac be forever plagued with an endless array of the maladies and malfunctions engendered by belief in their delusions? Again, there is no evidence to support this.

Belief may, in some way and to some degree, be necessary; but it is certainly not sufficient to induce a Placebo Effect. There must be something more. Perhaps something more primal. Let's step back and begin somewhere near the beginning, without preconceptions.

Ancient Greece

It is the second half of the fourth century B.C. A man "with no hair on his head" enters an Asclepian temple to undergo an "incubation," an Asclepian dream-healing. As the stone tablet (Stele I) outside the temple at Epidaurus would later proclaim: During that night's dream, the god anointed "his head with some drug" and "his hair grew."

What a quaint superstition, I thought upon first reading this account. After all, I understood that once baldness befell a man, it would take a reactivation of the genetic machinery inside the follicle cells to once again grow hair: transcription and translation, protein manufacture and extrusion. No minor matter. Certainly, I thought, something more powerful than the dream of an effete god's anointment must be required to reverse the cellular time machine. I smugly concluded that even though it was etched in stone, the Asclepian baldness cure did not happen.

Modern Times

Then, along came Minoxidil.

Minoxidil was originally cleared by the FDA for the treatment of high blood pressure. Unfortunately, it had a distressing side effect—hirsutism. I recall once examining a gentleman with a cough who had been taking Minoxidil for many months. As I lifted his shirt to auscultate his breath sounds, I was shocked to discover his back was densely covered with hair—no bare skin was visible anywhere.

The manufacturer was confronting a disaster. Desperately, they devised a placebo-controlled experiment. The test group would apply "the vehicle plus Minoxidil" to their bald scalps; the placebo group would apply the vehicle only. In other words, the test group got the drug while the placebo group got what medieval barbers called "snake oil" and the ancients called an anointment. The results were remarkable and rescued the manufacturer from financial ruin. Minoxidil (now, Rogaine™), caused hair to grow in 59% of men in the test group. Perhaps more remarkably, 33% (35.7% in a later report) of men in the placebo group—i.e., the "snake oil" group—also grew hair.

That quaint little Greek superstition no longer looks so quaint or little or superstitious, does it? The placebo worked: not quite as well as the drug, but with fewer risks. Perhaps the Minoxidil manufacturer should have trademarked the vehicle, Asclepia™ and sold it, too: "Proven in placebo-controlled clinical trials to work on one out of three men."

Nocebo Effects

In contrast to the aforementioned positive results, consider this startling report. In the *World Journal of Surgery* in 1983, patients with gastric cancer were treated after surgery with either placebo or one of two different chemotherapy regimens. All participants were given informed consent as to possible side effects, including hair loss. As expected, both chemotherapy groups experienced hair loss. What was astonishing was that in group A, the placebo group, 30.8% of patients also experienced hair loss!

This kind of outcome is referred to as the Nocebo Effect, meaning: an undesirable effect in the control group. Every placebo-controlled trial, in addition to demonstrating some degree of positive Placebo Effect, also demonstrates this nocebo phenomenon. Witness, for example, the plethora of negative symptoms (e.g., nausea, dizziness, vomiting, headache, etc.) present in the control group of most drug trials.

***

We have learned from the Greeks and the Minoxidil study that an idea (e.g., the dream of a god's anointment or a doctor's suggestion regarding an inert vehicle) can influence hair growth. Now we learn from the *World Journal of Surgery* that an idea (a doctor's "negative" suggestion regarding an inert substance) can also influence hair loss. In other words, ideas can both help and harm. Once again, we see the door swings both ways.

The question is, what pushes that door? If not "belief," what is it that provides the impetus for ideas to actualize? As we will soon see, the essence of the Placebo/Nocebo Effect can be extracted from the three stories above, all of which involve: (1) the presentation of an idea (expressed or implied) by an Authority; and (2) a physical response (i.e., hair growth or loss).

Which prompts us to ask, "What is an Authority?"

The Power of Authority

Human infancy is a time of utmost helplessness and dependency. Without support and guidance, the human infant cannot survive. Our species, therefore, requires infants be hardwired to recognize and submit to a protective, succoring Authority. It is a primordial survival pattern, an instinct: The child is born, helpless and dependent; it scans, finds, submits, learns and survives. What does the child scan for? How does it recognize the Authority? The answer is simple, if somewhat surprising. The child scans for The One least uncertain.

Understand, **this instinctual pattern reactivates whenever the organism feels imperiled.** Patterns Persist. Just as a reunion with a long-lost high school friend can reignite previous patterns of speech and play, so the return to helplessness and dependency reignites this prototypic quest for Authority. Moments in world history have triggered such collective quests: e.g., Pearl Harbor and 9/11. So too have moments in our own lives: natural disasters, emergencies, illnesses. What must be understood by professional caregivers is that the patients they serve often come with the urgent hunt for Authority fully activated. Their medical condition has rendered them helpless and dependent, or so they feel. Say what you will about the highly cognitive (and, therefore, late-evolutionary) topics of shared decision-making and selective paternalism, your patients—from a purely biological perspective—are seeking Authority and will recognize you as The One, provided you are The One least uncertain.

Again, to be clear, I am using Authority here as a defined term, meaning The One least uncertain. This is not a socially designated authority, such as a boss or a police officer. Rather, it is a biologically determined Authority, along the lines of a newborn's parent or a herd's Alpha.

Now, allow me this brief tangent:

"Sleep!"

It is early in my career. I am still under the influence of my university training (1976–79), during which medical paternalism was frowned upon, and interns and residents were strongly encouraged to share decision-making with their patients—whether patients asked them to do so or not. Any hint of authoritarian behavior was considered anachronistic.

Evening in the ED. A sudden blood-curdling scream. Around the corner whisks a gurney carrying a panicked young boy, his broken forearm grotesquely angulated. Beside him, his mother screams inconsolably. She is South American and speaks only a local dialect. It is unknown whether the boy speaks Spanish.

I immediately instruct Renee, my nurse, to get "Demerol, Stat." She vanishes around the corner. I am left with the distraught mother and desperate child. Patients and nurses on all sides are watching. I am in charge—white coat, stethoscope—The One least uncertain.

Earlier that month, I had asked a colleague of Dr. Ainslie Meares to show me how the great master had performed his famous nonverbal trance inductions. My friend, himself a renowned surgeon, demonstrated the technique. As I watched, I recall thinking "I'm never gonna use this, it's just too…peculiar."

Yet suddenly, my left hand extends to palm the young boy's head; my left thumb presses, with gradually increasing pressure, the center of his forehead. My breathing synchronizes with his. My right hand reaches out to the boy's shoulder, pressing down, as inarticulate grunts issue from somewhere deep inside me: medium pitch at first, then lower—as if a metaphor for "deeper." The boy's tears cease; his breathing regulates. "Duérmete!" I command ("Sleep!") He sleeps. I press down further on his shoulder, as if to convey "even deeper." Silence fills the room.

The mother is frozen, her mouth agape. Nurses' heads are cocked curiously. Patients gawk. "Um…just a little technique I learned," I say, almost apologetically. Renee returns, panting, syringe in hand. "Not necessary," I inform her. "Just press on his shoulder if he begins to wake." The boy sleeps through X-ray, reduction (i.e., straightening of the fracture) and casting. "I only had to press on his shoulder a couple times," Renee reports, proudly.

This one frozen moment mollified all my learnings about the stark evils of paternalism and forced me to reckon with **the power all healers possess.** The real decision is not whether to abandon the power of Authority, but rather how and when to best use it.

The case of that little boy with the forearm fracture inspired me to experiment. Here are just three examples of the stunning results I witnessed. There are hundreds more. As you read, realize "belief" did not feature prominently in any of these outcomes—neither belief by me nor belief by the patient. And yet…

The patient is in extreme respiratory distress—rapid labored breathing, intercostal muscle retraction, declining oxygen saturation. It is time to intubate (to place a flexible plastic tube in her trachea, connect it to a ventilator and assist her breathing). I guide the tube past her vocal cords...just a few inches to go. Then, resistance. A gentle push. More resistance, it will not pass. Normally, I would administer a muscle relaxant and/or push harder. This time, however, I decide to lean forward and whisper in her ear: "And it can enter like a breath of fresh air. Just let it. Just relax...and let it in...[the trachea relaxes, the tube advances]...and enjoy some deep easy breathing...that's right."

And, this:

(I had agreed to perform a home delivery for my friend's second child.) "Push...Push...," the baby is almost here. As the head descends, I can feel there won't be enough room. Not good: episiotomy versus the risk of a tear. We are between contractions. I decide to place two fingers, one on either side of the posterior vaginal introitus: "You can feel this finger pressing down, can't you? [She nods.] And this finger? [Nods, again.]" I synchronize my breathing with hers. "And I want you to tighten here first...really tighten." She does, on the left only. "And now relax that one and tighten here." She does, on the right only. The contraction begins. "And now really relax them both. Just relax... that's right...." The introitus opens generously. The head crowns. One gentle push, "Congratulations, it's a boy!"

And, finally:

She is 80 years old and has arrived by paramedics in ventricular tachycardia, a potentially fatal arrhythmia. Her blood pressure is dropping. We don't have much time. I instruct my nurse to get lidocaine for IV administration. She briefly disappears. I introduce myself and quickly explain what is going on. The patient is terrified. Another nurse charges the defibrillator. The whirr of electricity. I say, "While the nurse is fetching the medicine, let me remind you, your heart knows how to...be..in..a..reg..u..lar..rhy..thm," my cadence a metaphor for a regular rhythm. "And I need you to...do that now."

The nurse returns. I place the needle through the side port of the IV tubing. "Wait," says the nurse, "Look!" The rhythm has returned to normal. Blood pressure rising. I administer the lidocaine, but for prophylaxis.

In each of these cases, I had to cast aside both my reluctance to sound authoritarian and my considerable doubt that mere words could possibly relax a trachea, widen a birth canal or convert a deadly dysrhythmia. And yet, in each case the idea I offered produced the desired effect.

Now ask yourself, if some random stranger (minus the white coat and stethoscope) had used the exact same words on the same patients, would the results have been the same? Most likely not. But why? The idea of relaxation, dilatation or normalization does not change depending on who offers it. An idea, is an idea. The proposition 2+2 = 4 holds, whether asserted by a genius or a jerk. However, when a patient regresses to the primal state of helplessness and dependency, **the source matters far more than the suggestion.**

A parent, for example, may be wildly mistaken about right and wrong, politics and religion, what is healthy and what is not; yet, the parent's ideas splice into the nucleus of their young child's psyche, uncontested by the budding machinery of thought and reason. True, once one attains the age of reason, doubt and disbelief can discredit or undermine previously inculcated ideas. But generally speaking, reason operates secondarily. **Acquiescence to Authority proceeds via unconscious, autonomic routes, which activate instinctively in response to helplessness and dependency.** It is as if desiccated by doubt, the helpless and dependent mind draws desperately from the well of certainty—slaked not by facts and findings, but by conviction.

Today, we have only to scan the globe for demagogues to see this Principle of Least Uncertainty still active in the human herd. Observing this, Bertrand Russell concluded: "The whole problem with the world is that fools and fanatics are always so certain of themselves, and wiser people so full of doubts." But the principle is not only active in politics. An honest look at our scientific communities reveals that even in these hallowed realms of skepticism, source often pre-empts subject matter. Most scientific disciplines have, at one time or another, been haltered by charismatic "thought leaders" whom history would later prove wrong. For example, during the last several decades we have witnessed errant submission to Authority in Psychology, Epidemiology, Medicine, Biology...and more. Why? Because, whatever our shared fantasies of sublimation, we *Homo sapiens* simply cannot escape our biological underpinnings: phylogenetically and ontogenetically, science comes late to the game. We all share the tendency, when triggered, to follow The One least uncertain.

Let's summarize. The condition of helplessness and dependency triggers in all of us an instinctive search for The One least uncertain. Once identified, The One is then vested with Authority: Their reality becomes our reality, their ideas become our ideas. Think of parents and their young children or demagogues and their undissuadable adherents. It is as if the ideas of the Authority flow without resistance into the subject's psyche, wherein those ideas become both operative and, to a large extent, insulated from conscious repudiation.

Back to Placebo

Understanding Authority allows us to understand placebo/nocebo. In ancient Greece, the Aesclepian priest was The One least uncertain, and the ailing supplicant thus became the vessel of his suggestions. ("If you indulge in the ritual hymns and sacrifices, and fall asleep in the sacred *abaton*, then the god himself will visit and cure you.") During the Minoxidil clinical trial, the white-coated physician, keeper of the cure, was The One. ("If you smear this goo on your balding pate, then your hair will grow.") For the desperate cancer patients in 1983, the doctor who explained the risks and benefits of "the real drug" was the Authority. ("If you submit to this possibly curative treatment, then your hair will fall out.")

Throughout history and around the world today, Authorities (from shamans to surgeons) induce Placebo Effects with the same essential suggestion, which I call the "**Generic Placebo Suggestion**": "If you submit to X—this ritual/treatment, then Y—you will experience the prescribed outcome." And so long as, within the context of the culture, the intervention X is (1) credible at the outset, (2) somewhat difficult to achieve, but achievable, and (3) credible upon completion—a Placebo/Nocebo Effect (Y) will result. Not in everyone, but generally in 25–35% of patients.

Belief, it turns out, does matter. But it is not belief, whether by patient or caregiver, in the treatment or the outcome. It is, instead, the patient's belief in the Authority, the source. **So long as the patient believes in you (i.e., considers you The One least uncertain), your words have the power to hurt or heal.** And to be clear, I am not speaking only of psychological effects, like pain or analgesia. I am also speaking of so-called organic outcomes.

This final illustration says it all:

You're A Survivor—My Mother-in-Law, Michele

She is the linchpin of the entire family. Without her there would be no merry Christmas, no happy Thanksgiving, no loud and crazy Italian family dinners. Her diagnosis is Stage 4 ovarian cancer, one of the most dreaded and frightening diagnoses a woman can receive. We are all in the examining room with her, the whole worried family. We know "the odds."

She sits in her paper gown at the edge of the examining table, facing the door through which the surgeon (whom she hasn't met) will enter. A tremulous silence fills the room.

A white-coated Dr. Mark Wakabayashi opens the door, reading the chart as he enters. A half-step in, he looks up, gasps and exclaims: "You're a survivor!"

The rest is a fantastic blur: Something about…sometimes he can just tell, the surgery, lesions, debulking, timing, assistants, anesthesia…. None of it matters. "You're a survivor!" proclaimed by the surgeon who

*would open her abdomen and work seven focused hours to save her life.
"You're a survivor!" resounding like the peal of a thousand trumpets off
the marble walls of eternity. "You're a survivor!"*

*It is now 10 years since that fateful day. She IS a survivor. Each and
every holiday has been redolent with the aromas of her cooking,
the sounds of thundering grandchildren and the hearty laughter of
those who were with her when three words from a surgeon's mouth
lifted them all.*

P.S. Her "odds" of survival were 100%.

Summing Up

"Why today?" The answers to this question suggest unconscious ideas can often be contributory causes of illness. It is not just cells and molecules. It is also the emergent property of mentation that guides the whole organism.

The door swings both ways—these considerations further suggest that ideas can be contributory causes, not only to illness, but also to health and healing.

Placebo-controlled trials extinguish the "maybe" of mental causation by demonstrating that thousands of patients observed over decades of study stand as proof that ideas influence both physical and psychological outcomes.

Finally, **Placebo and Nocebo Effects** affirm the power of what I am calling **Authority** to push the door both ways—meaning, toward positive outcomes (e.g., hair growth, hemostasis, health) and negative outcomes (e.g., hair loss, pain, illness). Therefore, recognizing the influence of **Authority** in our daily practice, and learning to use it wisely, is fundamental to the Exquisite Art of Caregiving.

*"To attempt to predict anything beyond the relevant
horizon is futile—it is prophecy...."*

—David Deutsch, *The Beginning of Infinity*

Chapter 3:
FIRST, NO HARM

"**You** have a 90% chance of dying from this disease."

"**You** will likely have pain for a couple weeks."

"**You** will just have to learn to live with this."

UNDERSTANDING THAT AUTHORITY CAN COMPEL negative (as well as positive) outcomes, renders misstatements like those above especially vexing to practitioners of the Exquisite Art. All three are negative suggestions, all three are curses capable of doing harm.

In this chapter, we will explore why these misstatements are wrong and how to correct them. Once we have those understandings, we will also ask: Why do caregivers so often speak this way? Why are so many curses uttered so often, each and every day?

The Nature of Statistical Information

*I remember once asking my friend Skip, a gynecological surgeon,
how his day was going. "Tough," he said. "I just got done sitting down
with a 65-year-old lady with a large osteosarcoma in her pelvis.
Horrible prognosis. I had to tell her: 'Ruth, you have an 81% chance of
dying from your tumor.' But what could I do? I had to be honest."*

Honest? To be honest with this poor lady would have required two attributes my friend Skip did not exhibit that day: (1) knowledge about the nature of his information; and (2) the wisdom to deliver that information properly. First, let's look at the facts, then let's consider how best to present them.

The gold standard in evidence-based medicine is the RCT—randomized (controlled) clinical trial. In such trials, a sample of the general population is randomly assigned to receive either the experimental treatment/intervention or the placebo control. Ideally, neither the subjects nor the experimenters know who is receiving what (i.e, the protocol is "double-blinded"). The central notion here is that done right the results of an RCT can be extrapolated to individuals in the general population.

We have already discussed the important lessons RCTs teach about placebo—namely, that on average about 25–35% of people in an RCT will respond to placebo with physical (e.g., lower blood pressure, lower blood glucose, fewer kidney stones, etc.) and/or psychological (e.g., pain relief, nausea, headache, etc.) effects. These outcomes are driven by Authority—an instinctive acquiescence, at times of helplessness and dependency, to The One least uncertain.

We now need to focus on the notion of a "sample." This goes to the very heart of what it is an RCT can teach. In this respect, our principal concern is whether the study population in an RCT is ever representative of the individual patient who sits, helpless and dependent, before you.

First, let's consider how certain subpopulations relate to an RCT sample of the general population. Consider, for example, the early studies on hypertension. Generally, these studies involved adult males, often veterans. Is it logical to extrapolate the teachings of such an RCT to, say, African-American females? It is not, at least not without first proving that in respect of the study outcomes African-American females respond in a manner akin to the sample population. Or consider, the early studies of coronary artery disease, which also involved primarily middle-aged white males. Is it proper to extrapolate from those studies to, say, females, or Asians, or nonagenarians? Again, no—not without some kind of proof that such an extrapolation is accurate. Whenever the group under consideration does not "match" the selection parameters of a study (e.g., gender, race, age, concurrent medical conditions, etc.), extrapolation to that group is tenuous—often, more a leap of faith than a legitimate application of science. Fortunately, in recent years, more focus has been placed on this kind of discordance, and clinicians are tending toward greater care in extrapolating from a circumscribed study population to unmatched groups. The lesson is obvious: testing one group does not necessarily yield information about another group—not unless all the relevant variables are either "controlled for" or somehow (using, say, the new methods of causal inference) proven irrelevant.

What about extrapolating from the study sample to the individual patient who now sits before you? Let's return to Dr. Skip's patient with the osteosarcoma and assume that all parameters addressed in the study he has in mind match his patient: same gender, race, age, concurrent medical conditions, medications, occupational exposures, etc. In that study, 81 out of 100 patients died within two years of being diagnosed with the condition. What do we know? What knowledge do we possess that can be accurately shared with our patients?

"You have an 81% chance of dying from this condition."

Or, better:

"You have a 19% chance of surviving this condition."

While the latter is preferred, is it even accurate? Is either of these two statements really true?

The Fallacy of Extrapolation

What if your patient is somehow genetically advantaged with respect to immune defenses against the condition? Science may not have advanced sufficiently to ascertain this: in fact, it may be years before this genetic advantage is thoroughly understood. Does the RCT sample then speak to your patient's potential outcome? For example, was such a hidden variable even known or considered in the osteosarcoma study? Perhaps, all of the 19% who survived possess this currently unidentifiable mutation. Under those circumstances, if your patient has the mutation, she has a 100% chance of survival. This is entirely possible; and yet, as she sits before you, you presently have no way of knowing. Or, what if your patient is undergoing alternative treatments that were not controlled for in the sample population: for instance, treatment of contributing psychological causes, or selected supplements with the potential to forestall disease progression, or certain herbal remedies, or near-infrared laser treatments, or a host of other incompletely studied interventions that may have either positive or negative effects on the condition in question. Can you, then, reasonably extrapolate from the study population directly to your patient?

You cannot. Not with any certainty.

The key point here is that RCTs give you knowledge about the group under study. You can and often do make diagnoses and treatment choices based on the RCT's conclusions. But in making such decisions, it is important to recognize the limitations of your knowledge and the conjectural nature of your extrapolations. Essentially you are saying: "I know how a certain group behaves (means, medians, standard deviations, etc.). Based on that behavior, I suspect you **might** behave similarly. And since I have no better information to operate on, I will assume for the time being that you 'match' the study group sufficiently for me to tentatively predict and monitor the effect of the study intervention on your condition."

This is modern medicine. This is what we do. And it has been a remarkably successful approach, by and large. But you must also acknowledge what you do not know and what you cannot know. You do not know whether your patient belongs within a standard deviation or two of the mean or median of the RCTs results. Perhaps, she does. Perhaps, she is an outlier. You cannot know in advance, and therefore, beware the **Fallacy of Extrapolation**.

In this regard, a simple linguistic distinction can be immensely helpful, allowing Artful Caregivers to speak honestly while avoiding curses. It is the distinction between "you" and "some people, some patients, others." The former term, "you," is referred to by linguists as a specific referential index; the latter terms are called general referential indices. The former is a spear, the latter are shields.

"**You** have an 81% chance of dying" or "**You** have a 19% chance of surviving" are both untrue, because the statistical information on which these expressions are based does not inform you about an individual (i.e., **You**): no more than the temperature, pressure or volume of a gas informs you about the location or motion of any one molecule within that gas.

Here is the truth, Artfully delivered:

> *"Ruth, before I share your diagnosis, let me tell you the one thing I know from experience with absolute certainty. In medicine, miracles happen every day. I know this, and I know as I look at you that you may very well be the next miracle I witness.*
>
> *"Your diagnosis is osteosarcoma, which is a kind of cancer. And we all know that cancer is not a diagnosis we want. **Some people** die from this. But it is also a diagnosis, **Ruth, you can survive**. In fact, in scientific studies 19% of people (almost one in five) with this diagnosis do go on to beat it…and survive. People, perhaps, very much **like you**.*
>
> *"We will start treatment right away, and I'll be with you throughout. **Some people** can have difficulties with the treatment [list those]. But then, **Ruth, you** can also have a very smooth and comfortable course through treatment.*
>
> *"We will be together. Let's see **how well you do**."*

You have told her the truth: her diagnosis, treatment plan, and worst-case scenario. You have also told her that miracles do happen (which they do), and that she can be one of them. She can survive. This too is true. Your own data confirm it (19%).

What you have not done is pretend you know Ruth matches all the relevant characteristics of the RCT study group from which you are drawing your information. And, you have used the proper "referential indices" to convey both the facts and their associated uncertainties.

Had Dr. Skip used only this much of the Exquisite Art in his delivery, Ruth would have departed his office with a sense of hope and alliance. Moreover, given the profound Authority Dr. Skip held in this circumstance, isn't it also reasonable to suppose that his implicit survival suggestions would have carried at least a 25–35% chance of producing a more positive outcome?

The Fallacy of Prophecy

You also have not predicted Ruth's future. Nor should you. When a patient asks: "How much time do I have?" the answer is never, "You have…." There are two reasons for this. The first, we have already discussed: you simply cannot know how well or how poorly your individual patient matches the group whose information you are referencing. The "mean survival" pertains only to the group; it is not predictive of any one individual. The second reason is this: You cannot know the future. A cure for Ruth's condition, for example, could be discovered tomorrow or within the next two years. This is not at all far-fetched. In fact, it just happened in my own experience.

The Advent of Immunotherapy

My dear friend, Charlene—a 68-year-old female smoker—has just been diagnosed with non-small cell lung cancer with metastases to the brain. This is a terrifying diagnosis. Her oncologist has advised her, "These metastases are like ticking time bombs. We need to irradiate them immediately, then hit them with chemotherapy, and then surgically remove whatever remains in the brain."

Charlene asked my opinion. Not long before her inquiry, I had been reading the remarkable new studies on "immune checkpoint inhibitors." In a significant proportion of patients in the study samples, people with Charlene's tumor type had experienced a partial or complete disappearance of the tumor and its metastases. Knowing the dangers of radiation and chemotherapy, I told Charlene that if it were me, I would begin treatment with one of the new immunologic drugs—the checkpoint inhibitors. "I'm certain it is only a matter of time before these become the first-line treatment for your tumor type."

Charlene went with what her Authority-oncologist advised— namely, the standard of care. Her tumor did recede somewhat with chemo and radiation, but soon it began growing again. Fortunately, Optivo™ (an immune checkpoint inhibitor) then became available as a second-line drug. After Charlene's first dose of Optivo™, the tumor began to disappear. By the third dose, all that remained was a single brain metastasis.

Miraculous!

But that brain "met" appeared to be growing. The "ticking time bomb" metaphor had stuck in Charlene's consciousness. So, when the neurosurgeon said, "If it gets any bigger it will be harder to remove. We should go in now and get it out," Charlene agreed and the metastasis was removed. To both the surgeon's and Charlene's surprise, the pathology report indicated a mass devoid of living tumor cells and teeming with activated killer T-cells. The cancer had, in fact, been destroyed.

Though Charlene is recovering from some slight neurologic residua, she is alive and active to this day. It has been over three years and counting.

New treatments and cures are surfacing all the time. Regardless of how remote you believe the possibility, why deprive your patient of that hope?

But beyond the possibility of a new treatment or cure, there lies another cause for hope. It is, as I have already asserted, miracles happen. I will have much more to say on the patient/caregiver relationship in Chapter 8, but for now:

Miracles Happen

Althea is a buoyant 33-year-old female with an 8-inch-wide, biopsy-proven pelvic lymphoma. Owing to a chance meeting with an Indian guru, who told her, "You will be cured," she is uncommonly optimistic. But it is 1998, and the tumor is huge. The "prognosis" is grim.

She comes to see me for hypnosis, while her biopsy wound is healing, just before commencing chemotherapy. "I really think you can help me," she says. And, though I am privately far less optimistic than she, after six sessions her tumor is gone.

Her oncologist, a friend of mine, calls: "What have you done with Althea?" she demands.

"Just some positive suggestions," I say somewhat defensively, not yet knowing the outcome.

"Well," she continues, "We've done CAT scans and PET scans... and that tumor is gone. I'm presenting Althea to Tumor Board next Tuesday—miraculous!"

You may say this is a rare case of spontaneous remission. Perhaps. Though I've seen the same outcome with a Stage IV lung cancer patient. And I have had several patients with various cancers outlive their doctors' predictions by 5, 10 and even 12 years. Regardless, informing a patient that miracles happen and that new cures may come is like boring an airshaft to a trapped miner and delivering the oxygen of hope and the light of possibility.

There will never be a randomized controlled trial on miracles, yet they are as real as Charlene and Althea.

Humility

Avoiding inadvertent curses, as we have seen, entails a constant awareness of the nature and limitations of statistical information and the unpredictability of the future. This knowledge and wisdom deters us from the **Fallacies of**

Extrapolation and Prophecy and allows us to convey accurate information and positive suggestions without compromising our patients' needs for hope and alliance.

This seems simple, really. So why is it so rare?

The answer lies in the daunting challenge confronting all caregivers. Our task is impossible. And we know it.

Bertrand Russell long ago foresaw that as the universe of human knowledge continues to expand, and the mental capacity of the individual remains finite, specialization becomes inevitable. We now have specialists and microspecialists: cardiologists, electrophysiologists, neurologists, hepatologists, oncologists, immunologists and so on. Yet, before us sits not a heart nor a brain, not a liver nor a cell, but rather a whole individual: a patient replete with wants and woes, worries and wishes. How can we, with our finite expertise, ever succeed in the face of such overwhelming complexity?

> *One of the most challenging tasks in modern medicine is reading a plain chest x-ray. The shadow of an intricate three-dimensional structure (the human thorax) is cast on a monotone two-dimensional film, with objects and artifacts overlapping and obfuscating. Tomorrow morning, in a quiet room away from the racket and mayhem of the Emergency Department, a well-rested radiologist, coffee cup in hand, will study the film and render his reasoned interpretation. But that is tomorrow morning. Now, the Emergency Physician—with seven other patients clamoring for his or her urgent attention—must decide: Is the middle third (the "mediastinum") of this x-ray widened or not? Someone's life depends on it. The x-ray is of a 60-year-old hypertensive man with sudden excruciating substernal chest pain. His cardiogram suggests coronary artery occlusion (i.e., a heart attack), but the medication necessary to relieve the occlusion (i.e., a thrombolytic) could kill him if, instead of a heart attack, his aorta is dissecting (meaning,*

splitting apart). A widened mediastinum, wherein the aorta is located, would suggest the latter.

It is a small community hospital, miles from a more sophisticated facility. Time is of the essence. There are no other tests available to ascertain the diagnosis.

But here is the quiet truth: No Emergency Physician can read a plain chest X-ray as well as a radiologist. And no Emergency Physician can be 100% correct in discerning a widened mediastinum. This mistake is inevitable. Somewhere, at some time, under urgent conditions, with a patient writhing and anguish in the air, an Emergency Physician will elect to administer a blood-thinning thrombolytic medication to someone whose aorta is dissecting. And that patient will die of internal bleeding.

Knowing this, how do Emergency Physicians get up each day and drive to work—toward the inevitable collision of their high intentions and hopeless fallibility? And for that matter, how do surgeons "scrub in" knowing a welter of unmapped anomalies most surely awaits? Or psychiatrists, despite their list of labels and pallet of pills: how do they feign aplomb each day before the indecipherable madness that assails them from the couch? Or Chi-Gong Masters, before the impervious mass erupting from their patient's breast? Or chiropractors before the defiant limb? Or the mighty shamans before ineluctable death itself?

Failure haunts all healers.

And so, we puff up. We inflate. Not consciously, but as with most defense mechanisms, unconsciously. Our egos, like balloons, bloat with the hot air of hubris and only then rise to carry us over the abyss of self-doubt.

"He thinks he's a god," murmur his assistants. Indeed. What other way to face the looming blunders?

And then, from our patients, the questions come: "How long do I have?"

"What will happen next?" "What are my odds?" "Why me?"

And the answers: "You have two years at best." "You will probably have nausea and vomiting." "You have a 20% chance of survival." "Why you? Because you have a genetic mutation." Perhaps not the answers our patients had wished for. But answers nonetheless, answers an Authority is expected to know—betraying nothing of the doubt and uncertainty below.

Nothing exquisite here. Certainly, no art. Just simple human frailty.

While understandable, defensive puffery is not an acceptable strategy for caregivers. We see in the answers above how it produces false certainties that deflate and defeat our patients' best hopes. We also see how it forces disingenuousness and distance. The illusion of infallibility is an easy antidote to the potential paralysis of self-doubt, but a poisonous one.

Remember, Authority is instinctively conferred on The One least uncertain: that does not necessarily mean The One devoid of all doubt. Knowing where uncertainty lies insures us against deluding ourselves and our patients. Again, no one can foresee the course of any individual's recovery or decline—though we can influence it positively or negatively with salutary or deleterious suggestions. And no one can predict the future, especially as it relates to possible new discoveries and treatments. This knowledge of what we do not know—paired with the recognition that you can only do your best in any given moment, that mistakes are inevitable, and that forgiving those errors in advance is the best remedy—informs an empowering Humility that enables caregivers to truthfully impart hope to Ruth and Charlene and all the other patients whose trust in us is our most sacred charge.

When asked to predict the outcome of a patient with a dire diagnosis, the only right answer is: "I don't know. But what I do know is this:

"Miracles happen every day…[offer an anecdote]."

"While perhaps not the diagnosis we would have hoped for, people like

you do survive this condition…[offer statistical information—and tell it right]."

"*This is the course I recommend, based on my best knowledge at this time…[subject to change, as I continue to study the evolving research].*"

"*And I will be with you throughout. Let's see how well you do.*"

Humility, not hubris—a graceful bridge over the abyss of self-doubt.

Summing Up

Endowed with Authority, caregivers must learn to avoid negative suggestions. To achieve this, we need to beware the Fallacies of Extrapolation and Prophecy inherent in many of the common curses caregivers so often deliver. Remaining mindful of the nature of statistical information and the unpredictability of an individual's future can help us prevent careless misstatements. Additionally, we must confront head-on the daunting nature of our task and the fearful defenses we are reflexively prone to erect. In this regard, the wisdom to elevate humility over hubris will serve us well.

"The whole of science is nothing more than a refinement of everyday thinking."

—Albert Einstein

Chapter 4:

A REFINEMENT OF EVERYDAY COMMUNICATION

WE NOW TURN TO THE TASK of saying it right. The Exquisite Art of Caregiving requires that clinicians communicate with elegance and economy that maximizes the likelihood of achieving their intended outcomes. It doesn't matter whether those intended outcomes are mental or physical. The former might consist of responses such as compliance to a treatment regimen, agreement to undergo a procedure, or relief of pain or anxiety. The latter could include: hemostasis, joint reduction, accelerated wound healing, tumor shrinkage, or thwarted autoimmunity. The task of the caregiver is to persuade both mind and body.

What does matter is that our words and gestures convey what we intend and that our ideas are somehow empowered to actualize. In Chapter 2, we learned that our Authority as caregivers will drive at least some of our suggestions to actualization. For example, in placebo-controlled clinical trials, some 25–35% of patients will generally respond to our ideas, expressed or implied. Those ideas, as we also learned, can be either salutary or deleterious. Some patients will experience amelioration of their physical condition; some will suffer nausea and headaches; others will have both kinds of reactions. But, a

25–35% likelihood of compliance is hardly "exquisite." We need to learn how to enhance our persuasive powers, to increase the likelihood our suggestions will be realized.

Much of what follows derives from the world of hypnosis and, in particular, Neuro-Linguistic Programming (see Resources). And yet, as I learned in the Emergency Department—where there was often no time for trance induction or structured sessions—these skills and learnings apply as well to regular caregiver conversations. Think of what follows as a refinement of everyday communication: a way of presenting clear and precise ideas in a manner that increases the likelihood of their actualization. One caveat. As with any new skill—typewriting, bicycling, a new language—the initial learning phase entails conscious effort and concentration. It takes some work. The lessons that follow will require your active engagement. However, like those other skills, habits form quickly, and the phase of focused concentration soon gives way to unconscious fluidity. Skillful and effective communication rapidly becomes second nature.

My advice is to proceed at your own pace. Begin by adding one and then another of the elements discussed below. Soon enough, you will have incorporated all of the elements, and the astounding results of your efforts will have begun to accrue.

The Red Ball

Let's begin with a simple thought experiment. Your task is to convince as many volunteers as possible to picture a red ball. Trivial? Not really. Remember the painless injection technique I outlined in Chapter 1? Directing someone to "just look" or "just listen" is often all it takes to induce momentary anesthesia. And from painless injections, it is only a few small steps to painless procedures and other salutary outcomes.

Even more important, as you'll see in the next chapter, the lessons you take from this simple "Red Ball" exercise will carry into virtually every patient/ caregiver conversation you have for the rest of your career. How to offer an idea and have it accepted and acted upon—this is the essence of the Exquisite Art of Caregiving. This is where the magic begins.

Direct Suggestions

Let's imagine a large room filled with healthy students who have volunteered for an experiment. Without prelude, you enter the room and demand:

> *"Picture a red ball!"*

This is an unadorned direct suggestion. A mandate.

It is possible, especially if you are perceived as something of an Authority (perhaps, a professor) that roughly 25–35% of the subjects will comply and envision a red ball. In essence, this is akin to a Placebo Effect. However, the remaining 65–75% will not respond, either because they are: (1) pre-occupied or distracted with other thoughts and activities, (2) resistant to your questionable authority (e.g., "who does he think he is?"), or (3) both.

Interestingly, our simple thought experiment has already yielded a valuable lesson. To be broadly persuasive, we need to:

1. focus our subject's attention; and
2. avoid their resistance.

Focusing Attention

For our purposes, let's consider consciousness or attention (I will use these terms interchangeably) as being somewhat like a flashlight, whose single illuminating beam can splay, forming several beams, and coalesce. Whatever the light shines upon, we are conscious of—whether external, like the words on this page, or internal, like thoughts or dreams. The flashlight can be controlled by the one experiencing consciousness or by someone else. And that someone else can be a caregiver, a sage, a storyteller, etc.

The question now becomes: How do we focus the divergent beams of our volunteers' consciousness into a single beam and then direct it to PICTURE A RED BALL?

Confusion Focuses Attention

Just as Nature abhors a vacuum, so Mind abhors confusion. The instant confusion occurs, the divergent beams of consciousness converge into a single focused beam, searching for resolution. You may be resting peacefully, for example, at a seaside bar, listening to the surf, feeling the fresh sea breeze, aware of the scent of the sea and the sight of gulls wheeling overhead. Suddenly, a violent crash booms behind you! Gone is the surf, the breeze, the scents and sights. Your attention now focuses, searching for the source of the commotion. "What just happened?" The once peaceful splay of consciousness has urgently converged to resolve the confusion.

We can make good use of this phenomenon in our "Red Ball" experiment by realizing **any time a question is raised, it provokes momentary confusion.** Ask a question and the beam of consciousness converges until the answer is found. Knowing this, instead of beginning with a direct suggestion to an inattentive crowd, you might instead begin with: "How many of you volunteers already understand how you can win in this experiment and the potential benefits of winning?" Now, you are gathering their attention. But just to be sure, you might add: "And, wouldn't it be great if you could all be winners?" Of course, you will have to hold their attention. Often this is achieved by peppering the conversation with frequent questions, as is the custom in everyday British conversation: "Isn't it?"

Pattern Interruption

Pattern interruption is another reliable way to provoke confusion and thereby focus and hold attention. Here are two simple methods you can readily intersperse in your daily patient/caregiver conversations to focus and maintain your patient's attention.

1. Longer than usual...pauses. (sic)

Often, I take a long, contemplative breath during such a pause.

EXAMPLE: "Now, I'd like you to...[deep, thoughtful breath] __ **follow these instructions.**"

2. Violating syntax

While there are a variety of syntactic violations that can be used (many of which I will share later on), here are the two I use most often.

A. Dropping the "to" in the infinitive: to do, to be…etc.

EXAMPLE: "Now, I'd like you __ **follow these instructions.**"

B. Splitting the infinitive and inserting the subject's proper name in between.

EXAMPLE: "Now, I'd like you to, **John, follow these instructions.**"

These structures often, as here, perform the dual function of both focusing attention and disguising a mandate (*in bold*).

As a caregiver, you often have the attention of your charge or patient by virtue of your Authority. Yet, there are times when they may be distracted or when you may wish to give particular emphasis to your words. At such times, these simple measures can be instrumental.

> EXAMPLE: *"Have you ever wondered why some patients don't just…*
> *[deep breath]…, **John, follow the doctor's advice?** I do. Maybe they*
> *don't realize how easy it is __ **get well.**"*

Asking questions and utilizing brief pattern interruptions, simple as it seems, allows you to draw in and focus your patients' attention. After that, you have only to avoid their resistance in order to succeed.

***

Back to our thought experiment. Imagine you now begin as follows:

> *"Who here wants to succeed at this potentially enriching experiment?*
> *Good. And, along those lines, how many of you…[deep breath]…find*
> *it easy __ PICTURE A RED BALL? Just curious." (sic)*

I guarantee this construction will draw far more attention than the previous mandate.

Avoiding Resistance

Now, let's turn to our second task: avoiding resistance. Once someone starts to resist, the unproductive pattern of contrariness commences. And, Patterns Persist. A moment's skepticism can become an abiding distrust. The Exquisite Art requires that we avoid resistance, so as to commence a different, more productive pattern.

In this regard, so-called permissive language was one of Dr. Milton Erickson's greatest gifts to caregivers. Erickson discovered how to engage even the most obstinate patient, by cleverly sidestepping both conscious and unconscious resistance. We will learn much more about this remarkable healer and his methods in later chapters. For now, it is crucial to understand that for all its elegance and nuance, Dr. Erickson's permissive language basically boils down to one simple rule—speak incontrovertibly: meaning, in a manner that cannot be denied or disputed. Far better this than the contentious talk of an authoritarian. For if a patient cannot disagree with you, the pattern of agreement commences.

Here are some essential rules for **Permissive Language**:

1. Avoid Mandates

This ironic request is an easy habit to cultivate. When talking with patients, it is best to refrain from using the strongly insistent words "will" or "must." For example, I once overheard a surgeon declare: "When you wake up, the pain WILL be excruciating." "The hell it will," thought the patient, as I later learned when he sought more comforting suggestions through presurgical hypnosis.

Instead of "will" or "must," it serves to use words that allow for other possibilities: words like "can, could, may, might." These words imply their opposites (cannot, could not, may not, might not), and so are much more difficult to resist. "Some patients MIGHT experience discomfort upon waking," is far better than "You will experience excruciating pain." The former honestly conveys the possibility of pain, without imparting a negative suggestion.

These are the kinds of subtle linguistic turns that, while relatively easy to incorporate, distinguish the Exquisite Art from potentially harmful, haphazard speech.

The other word to avoid is "don't." Why? First, because it readily provokes resistance, as any parent of an adolescent will tell you. Second, because in order to make sense of "don't do it," you must first understand the doing of it, and then negate that. Imagine a child is precariously carrying a slightly over-filled glass of milk across a beautiful new carpet. You can either shout, "Don't spill the milk!" or calmly observe, "Tommy, that's a good way to HOLD your glass and KEEP it level." Instead of "don't," it almost always works to substitute "hold" or "keep," and then turn the phrase to the positive.

2. Indirect Suggestions

A far more effective approach than mandates (except in rare instances) is the use of indirect suggestions. Here are three widely applicable examples that apply easily to everyday caregiver conversations. Let's see how they might work in our Red Ball experiment:

A. "I wonder…."

"I wonder if winning in this experiment will have anything to do with your ability to PICTURE A RED BALL."

Notice how much more difficult it is to resist my personal wondering than the previous direct command?

B. "I don't need to tell you…."

"I don't need to tell you how useful a visual imagination can be. After all, those who can PICTURE A RED BALL might have a real advantage. Right?"

Here if someone choses to resist, they will have to say: "Yes, you do need to tell me…."

C. Quotes

Again, it is hard to resist the mere recollection of someone else's words.

"All I know is some professor was overheard this morning saying, 'If you can PICTURE A RED BALL, you can win.'" Indirection, as you can see, is a deft way of conveying an idea without provoking resistance or resentment. Let's put these three methods of indirection together in a commonly encountered clinical scenario, and see how they differ from the usual manner of presenting the information:

> *"I'm sure I don't need to tell you that the health risks of obesity are substantial. Yet, I wonder what it would take for someone to inspire you to follow a healthier lifestyle? Most of my patients say: 'If my own child told me they needed me to be around for my grandchild's graduation.' Or something like that. And yet, everyone's different. Some people wait a week or two before the urgency finally...[pause]...hits you."*

We all know what a direct suggestion to adopt a healthy lifestyle or quit smoking would likely have achieved—conscious resistance and, possibly, resentment. It reminds me of Herman Hesse's famous line: "Unfortunately, commandments have always had a catastrophic effect on me." He is not alone.

Here is an actual example of how effective indirection can be:

Mr. Two-Pack

He is a two-pack-a-day man. "Damn cough" is his chief complaint. I've taken his history, examined him and checked his X-ray. The diagnosis is bronchitis. As usual, the ED is busy. Others are waiting. I explain the diagnosis and treatment briefly, hand him a prescription and walk out the door—almost.

One step out, I turn around as if having forgotten something and say: "By the way, sir, you know you don't need to stop smoking...today?" He nods quizzically, and I'm gone. The implication, of course, is you DO need to stop smoking someday.

Months later, I'm walking from the ICU back to the ED, and Mr.
Two-Pack stops me. "Doc, Doc... Do you remember me?" he asks,
explaining he is there to visit a friend in the ICU. "You did something
to me. I just know you did. What was it?" He explains that shortly
after I had treated him, he suddenly stopped smoking. Couldn't say
why. All he knows is it was something I had done.

"Isn't it amazing how some things can have lasting effects?" I say
(never missing an opportunity to embed an indirect suggestion). "Now,
sir, if you'll excuse me," I continue, "I have to get back to the ED."

Impressive. And yet, indirection doesn't always work. Sometimes your influence needs to be even more subtle. Enter the metaphor.

> NOTE: For our purposes, the distinction between metaphor and simile, or allegory and parable, is splitting semantic hairs. Either way, we are telling a story to which the patient, consciously and or unconsciously, attaches meaning.

3. Metaphorical Suggestions

Have you ever noticed how virtually all sages, when asked a question, respond with a story? I was fortunate to have Share K. Lew, a Taoist priest and grandmaster, as a dear friend for almost 30 years. When I would ask for his thoughts on some challenging aspect of my life, he would usually answer with a story. And since the story was meant as a metaphor, its truth (in the non-fiction sense) was less important than its meaning. Here, wisdom trumps veracity. Moreover, a good story, like a brilliant novel, will have different meanings to different listeners at different times.

For example:

As a surfer in my 30's, I struggled with the conflict between my desire
to compete for waves at the best spots and my wish to experience the
peacefulness and serenity of the sea. "What shall I do, Sifu [meaning,
Teacher]?" I asked.

He told me: "A young priest I knew, skilled in martial arts, once encountered a hunched old man on a narrow path through the rice fields. 'Stand aside old man,' commanded the arrogant youth. The old man would not yield. 'I said, stand aside!'

Still, the old man stood his ground. Angry, the young priest pushed the old man. But, like a granite boulder, he could not be moved. Again and again, the infuriated young priest pushed this way and that— always to no avail. The young priest's efforts were like a soft breeze against a mighty mountain. At length, the frustrated youth rolled up his pants and trudged around the old man through the mud."

Sifu explained that in those days there were still a few surviving practitioners, like the old man, of the ancient Chi-Gung arts. Himself old and thin, Sifu concluded: "You never know who knows what."

I'm sure this story means something different to each of you. And tomorrow it may take on yet another meaning. For me, as Sifu's story slowly sank in, I came to realize that since I could not move the crowd from the choicest surf spots, I would move myself by paddling south to enjoy solo-surfing on less shapely waves. I realize that to a non-surfer this may seem obvious or trivial, but at that time in my life, it was neither. The story brought peace where there was turmoil. Had Sifu said, "Doctor Steve, don't be stupid…just paddle south," I would have stubbornly concluded that a Taoist priest cannot possibly comprehend the depths of a surfer's dilemma.

Now, back to our Red Ball experiment. Following our opening questions and indirect suggestions, why not add a metaphor:

"I don't know if you people know this or not, but last year's winner was awarded a hot air balloon ride—which she loved. We all watched her climb in and lift off. It was a beautiful evening. Can you imagine? As the RED BALLOON rose higher and higher, we lost sight of her and the balloon's basket. Looking up, all that you could see was what

looked like a beautiful RED BALL. Can you picture that? A RED BALLOON floating high in the evening sky…"

This is a made-up story, about a volunteer (so the listeners will relate). I frequently begin my metaphors with, "I once had a patient who…" or "I once knew a man/woman who…" Erickson was the master of this approach—often couching a curative suggestion in the story of "a patient" who had once achieved an outcome analogous to his current patient's goal. Sidney Rosen, M.D. has compiled a rich compendium of Ericksonian stories in his book entitled, *My Voice Will Go with You.* Sometimes, I alter one of these tales to suit the situation. Other times, I simply invent a story (beginning with, "Someone once said….") and weave the appropriate suggestions into it.

The Communication Continuum

As you can see, we are moving along the communication continuum—far from haphazard speech—and heading toward maximum persuasiveness. Once you have someone's attention, using permissive language is a masterful way of getting your ideas across.

If you think about it, these refinements make you more persuasive not only as a caregiver but also in all your everyday communications. Therefore, it makes sense to practice throughout the day, until these fundamental elements of the Art become second nature. I assure you, you will be as much the beneficiary of those efforts as will your patients.

***

Now, back once more to our Red Ball experiment.

If you are standing before an audience that regards you as an Authority, and you already have their complete attention, then "Picture a red ball!" is all you need to say. But, if you do not have the audience's complete attention, if they do not regard you as an Authority, then "Picture a red ball!" will, more likely than not, fail to evoke the desired response—at least, in the majority of people.

To elicit maximum cooperation, we need to refine our communication by first capturing people's attention and, then, offering suggestions without incurring their resistance. Imagine our volunteers' responses to our newly acquired skills:

You enter and ask:

> *"How many of you already…understand how to win in this experiment? Uh-huh. Wouldn't it be great if you all could win, and win big?"* **(Confusion—*created by asking questions—*focuses attention.)**

> *"Let me tell you a little secret. A professor I know was overheard this morning saying, 'If you can* PICTURE A RED BALL, *you will win.' Of course, I don't need to tell you how useful a visual imagination can be."* **(Quotes avoid resistance. "I don't need to tell you…" is an indirect suggestion.)**

> *"In fact, I distinctly remember one winner from a previous session telling her peers, "It's all about visual imagination. You just close your eyes and* PICTURE A RED BALL, *like a balloon floating in the sky, and the rest is easy."* **(A metaphor,** *about "one winner.")*

> *"So, I wonder if I could ask all of you to just close your eyes for a moment and allow yourselves…*PICTURE A RED BALL…*and just look. Really look. And when you see it, when you can* PICTURE A RED BALL, *raise your hands to signal your success…."* **("I wonder…"** *introduces an* **indirect suggestion.)**

In the next chapter, we will begin to apply these new refinements to everyday caregiving: offering curative suggestions, delivering informed consent, explaining diagnoses and treatment plans—all without provoking resistance or inadvertently instilling negative suggestions. I guarantee these simple tools will change the way you practice and the way your patients respond.

But before we jump to practical applications, there are two more techniques worth learning. The first involves our deeds, how we act and gesture; the second involves our words, specifically, what certain words really mean. It is as if we have just acquired some much-needed hand tools; now, let's add a couple of power tools.

Underscoring

How do you convey to a patient (in a manner that skirts resistance) that what you are now saying is exceptionally important? In our red ball experiment I CAPITALIZED the key suggestion: PICTURE A RED BALL. How do we convey the emphasis of those ALL CAPS, especially when the message is critical? The answer is you underscore it, by using either your eyes or your voice, or both.

This is a tremendously powerful technique that can be used virtually anytime you wish to place emphasis on an idea. During the UNDERSCORED communication, I use direct eye contact coupled with a barely perceptible strengthening of my voice. The rest of the time, I allow my eyes to look slightly down or to the side, using my normal voice or perhaps even a slightly softer tone.

For example:

> *It is 1988, before the blossoming of interventional cardiology—emergency angioplasty, selective thrombolysis, etc. I am at the bedside of a 56-year-old gentleman explaining to him that he has had a heart attack. He was treated as we treated most such patients at the time: oxygen, nitrates, low dose morphine, atropine for transient bradycardia (slow heart rate). No longer in pain, his cardiac rhythm normal, it is now time to talk. Soon he will be moved to the ICU.*

> *"In terms of prognosis, sir," my eyes locking with his only during the ALL-CAPS moments, as my voice in those same moments waxes subtly more forceful, "remember, the heart is a muscle. And ALL MUSCLES KNOW HOW TO HEAL. In fact, the healed part of a tissue is often EVEN STRONGER THAN THE ORIGINAL tissue." During the "lowercase moments," I would regard his wife across the bedside or place my*

hand above his heart and regard it. "So you can JUST RELAX and let your body do what it has so often done before…and knows how to do now…JUST SAFE AND COMFORTABLE HEALING."

An hour after the gentleman's transfer to the ICU, his graceful wife paid me a visit. "I don't quite know what you were doing there, doctor, or how you were doing it," she said. "But whatever it was, I could see him calming down as you were speaking. And once we got settled in the ICU, he turned to me and said: 'Honey, while that doctor was talking…I don't know…I just somehow knew this whole thing would work out fine.' So, thank you, Doctor," she said. "Thank you very much."

Gratifying? Definitely. We will never know from this one case whether the only effect of those underscored words was to instill in my patient a sense of ease about his recovery. Did his heart heal faster? Was his subsequent uneventful hospitalization a consequence? What we do know is that offering a layer of care beyond monitors and medications mattered enough to prompt a worried wife to briefly leave her husband's side and say, "Thank You."

I use UNDERSCORING all the time in clinical practice. It punches in the message, leaving no doubt in your patient's unconscious mind as to what really matters. When you were young, you might have been taught: "Look people right in the eye and tell it straight." Now we are refining that teaching: "Look people right in the eye WHEN IT MATTERS MOST and TELL IT SMART."

Linguistic Virtuosity
Artful Caregivers first learn the rules and then selectively break them with graceful audacity.

One such "rule," taught to me by various luminaries in the clinical hypnosis establishment, was "never use the word 'try' when attempting to elicit a response—e.g., 'try to relax.'" During my studies for the American Board of Medical Hypnosis, various mentors repeatedly hammered in this dictum. We sense intuitively there is something to it. Right? For example, as parents we become exasperated when, upon reminding our kids to keep their rooms clean, they respond with a snide, "I'll try." Turns out, our intuition has merit, but the rule is misconstrued. In fact, breaking this rule leads us directly into the realm of linguistic virtuosity and to a one-sentence trance induction for children.

But first, here is how this discovery came about. One day, I was reading an account in which Dr. Erickson was explaining a psychotherapy session he had conducted to a group of students, "You see," he said of the patient, "she used the word 'try,' and 'try' implies an obstruction." Suddenly, it was as though the nail my mentors had been hammering shot straight through the plank, leaving a hole in its place, through which poured in the bright light of understanding. **It's not about avoiding certain words, I realized. It's about knowing their meaning—their full meaning—and using that knowledge deliberately.** Almost instantly I thought, what if I say to a frightened child: "I want you to try...just try...to stay awake for one—no two—sorry, one more minute. Just try." The implied obstruction would have to be some overwhelming compulsion to sleep! The "one...two...one" would be confusing enough to gain and hold the child's attention, while at the same time putting a very short limit on their resistance. I couldn't wait to get to the ED and test it out.

Single-sentence Induction

She is nine years old. Scared before she arrived, she is even more scared now, with all the noise and suffering around. She has a deep finger laceration. Her mother sits by her side, doing her best to calm the child.

"And who is Alice?" I ask with feigned ignorance, having seen her name on the chart. (At least she isn't completely helpless; she knows something the doctor doesn't.) Alice raises her uninjured hand, meekly.

Now, I hold up first one finger, then two, then one again (continuing to slowly alternate) and say: "Now Alice, I wonder if you could TRY... just really TRY TO STAY AWAKE...for one [while having two fingers up]...um, I mean two [while showing one finger]...one more minute.

Just TRY TO STAY AWAKE." Upon which I signaled a gentle shh-sign to the mother. (Since the parent is the pre-eminent Authority, it always serves to enlist their cooperation.)

In seconds Alice went, as it were, to wonderland. Her eyes fixed in a distant gaze, she never flinched or whimpered or even knew what was happening as I repaired her laceration. At one point along the way I added: "…and wherever you are, you can just go from one comfortable happy place to another. Just happy and comfortable."

Mom was relieved. Alice, too. But I was triumphant. I have used that single-sentence induction, now, on hundreds of children. Always with success, except when I fail to silence the parent: "Sweetie, is the doctor hurting you?"

Again, the real rule isn't "avoid the word 'try.'" Rather it is: Know the meaning of your words, down to the nuances, and chose them deliberately.

Pearls

In addition to **"try,"** here are a few "Pearls" and their meanings. I use all of them, often; they are precious tools in the Exquisite Art. Of course, there are many more. What follows is simply a useful list of some of the most impactful.

1. Just

"Just," as we have discussed above, means— "and nothing more." When a patient JUST listens, or JUST watches, or JUST thinks…they are not feeling; their attention is fully absorbed in the auditory, visual or cognitive mode. In the Exquisite Art of Caregiving, NOT FEELING is frequently a good thing.

2. Really

"Do you know what that word means?" I ask. "Yes, I do," comes the reply. "Do you **really** know what it means?" "Really" casts doubt on the antecedent. This is a critically important word when it comes to the caregiver's task of discovery. Here is a classic example:

I have listened to the patient's history for an hour, assiduously taking notes, nodding assents, asking questions. When did you start smoking, who in your family smokes, how does smoking make you feel, what prompted you to see me?

Now comes the moment of truth, the only moment that actually matters in the first session:

"Very good, I think I understand, and let me thank you for being so forthright and honest about your smoking issues. But now I have to ask you what might actually be the most important question. And forgive me if it seems a bit awkward. But I really do need to know..."

The way I'm asking this is for two reasons: First, I am creating some preliminary confusion in order to focus attention; second, by dithering I am doing what Erickson called "building response potential." This means, I am teasing them, drawing them in, making them really curious about what I am about to ask, and causing them to be eager to answer.

*"So here is my question...Do you **really** want to quit smoking...now?" This, as you can sense, casts doubt on all the antecedent history and asks for the "real" truth.*

At this point, you as the caregiver must do something very difficult. Remember our, "Why today? Just guess" discussion. In that situation, it is important for you to stop speaking; wait out the silence, knowing the answer will come. Now, following "do you REALLY want to quit...now," you must stop listening. No matter what the answer, do not listen to it. Instead, just watch. Really watch: especially the patient's head movements.

If you do this keenly and honestly, you will see one of two responses. Either the patient will nod their head in an up-and-down assent, or the patient will shake their head in a back-and-forth dissent. A nonverbal "yes" or "no."

John Grinder calls this a "congruency check." Is the patient's unconscious intention congruent with their expressed wishes? Imagine how broadly applicable congruency checks are in the healing arts: "Do you understand? I mean, do you REALLY understand?"

Of course, in the above example, if the patient nods his or her assent you proceed with therapy. However, if their nonverbal message is "no," then you would be wasting your time and their money to proceed. Beginning practitioners of the Art often feel especially uncomfortable at this juncture: they have listened and related, invested their time and attention. They want to help and very likely believe they can help. Let me urge restraint. Trust me once, and thereafter your own experience will confirm and reconfirm the following:

> *"I hear you, but let me show you what you actually did while saying 'yes.'" Then, demonstrate the negative nonverbal response. "My experience tells me some deeper part of you is just not quite ready to quit. Now is just not the time. Right? But please know, if things change my door is always open for you."*

> *At this point, almost invariably, the patient will let out a sigh of relief: "Ah Doc, you're so right. Honestly, my wife has been on me relentlessly. To tell the truth, I need my cigarettes now…at least until things lighten up at work a bit." Or, something like that…REALLY.*

3. Even

"Even" implies the opposite of "Really": it affirms (rather than casts doubt on) the antecedent. For example: As you've been reading, you have probably already begun to see the value in refining your everyday communications. What I'm asking you to do now is…learn EVEN more.

Whenever you are attempting to elicit a response from a patient, like relaxation, it serves to follow the OBSERVE >> RATIFY >> AUGMENT pattern. In essence this turns you, the caregiver, into a biofeedback machine reinforcing desired responses.

"I wonder if you could allow your eyes to close…and gently relax."You observe the eyes slowly closing, the shoulders settling down. "Uh-huh [OBSERVE] >> that's right [RATIFY] >> even more [AUGMENT]."

Simple, and yet when employed by an Artful Caregiver, powerful. "Un-huh… that's right…**even** more."

4. Try

"Try," as noted in the introduction to this topic, implies an obstruction. I've already shared how this knowledge led me to a one-sentence trance induction for children. Let me share one more example of "try's" broad applicability, and then challenge you to find other clever uses. This is where the Art comes in.

As a prelude, some of you may need two bits of information: (a) "Oh say can you see, by the dawn's early light…" are the first words in the USA's national anthem. As such, almost all native-born U.S. citizens have known this phrase since childhood. Patterns Persist. (b) The goal is to get the patient to think the words: "see" and "light." I know that if they are fully focused (remember, confusion focuses attention) on the internal sound or thought of these words, they will not be attending to their feelings.

"Try to not say what I don't say. I know that's a bit confusing, so let me say it again, because it's important: Try to not say what I don't say."

You know enough now about the Art to understand that I now have their full attention. Next, for painless injections:

"Oh say can you __ [at this point, I insert the needle], by the dawn's early __ [now, I inject the medication, painlessly]."

Here, the word "try" connotes an obstruction to "not saying what I don't say." That obstruction, as it happens, directly opposes the tendency for patterns (in this case, the acoustic pattern of the national anthem) to persist. The patient cannot help but say, usually internally, the words "see" and "light." And while their complete attention is focused on trying not to say those words, the injection is given—again, painlessly.

5. *You vs. It*

We have already discussed the important distinction between the specific referential index "you" and the general referential index "some people, some patients, others." We now need to understand an additional distinction—this time between "**you**," as it refers to one's complex self-conception, and "**it**" as it refers to the non-Self rest of the world. Much of this knowledge comes from the realm of hypnosis, but as you'll see, it has critical applicability to many of our more common "non-trance" communications. For example:

> *"I've been working with meditation and affirmation to get rid of **my** cancer, but it just doesn't seem to be working," explained Clair, when I first met her.*
>
> *"Well, I'm sure you would agree that it is easier to remove a pest when you can see it than when it is camouflaged," I said.*
>
> *Clair cocked her head, quizzically: "Huh?"*
>
> *"Let's call the cancer what it is, so that we don't confuse your unconscious. Let's call it, THE CANCER, not 'my cancer.' It's a small but important distinction. That way, when we talk about you, we can talk about YOUR healing systems and YOUR cells and YOUR organs and YOUR hopes and dreams."*
>
> *"Oh, I see," she said, smiling. "Yes, let's do that. I hate that cancer; it's a pest and I want it gone from MY body."*
>
> *"Exactly, and so do I, Clair," I rejoined. "Shall we begin expelling IT?"*
>
> *"You bet," she said enthusiastically.*

In earliest infancy, we begin to piece together what eventually becomes a grand aggregate of agencies and experiences we call Self, and which we embrace with words like "me," "I," "mine," "my," etc. Other people, of course, refer to our Self with words like "you" and "your." Within this grand aggregate exist all the elements of body and mind that we have learned to command volitionally, experience consciously and envelop conceptually within our physical and mental Self.

In trance work, for example, if I call someone's hand "your hand," I am including it within their self-conception and hence within their volitional control; whereas, if I refer to their hand as "it" or "the hand," I have subtly dissociated it from Self, rendering it capable of non-volitional/non-ordinary behavior— the hallmark of so-called deep trance phenomena. For example, I can suggest that **the** "unconscious" will lift **the** hand—thereby evoking hand levitation. Then, I can use this lifted hand as: "…an example of how the unconscious can move thousands of cells, billions of molecules, octillions of atoms in response to a single idea…lifting a hand to help. And if the unconscious can do that, certainly it can move a few million T-cells to destroy that tumor…."

We are not studying trance work (not yet, anyway), but we can still learn some of its lessons. Grasping this important distinction between words connoting "Self" and words connoting "non-Self" contributes greatly to the avoidance of negative suggestions like these:

> *Your infection is a stubborn one.…*
>
> *Your tumor is an aggressive cell type.…*
>
> *Your disease is one we will just have to…*
>
> *Your pain is not likely to…*

These curses inject the ailment into your patient's self-conception like a mosquito injects malaria into its victim's bloodstream. Since our job is often to extirpate suffering or disease, why not begin with a simple linguistic excision: **the** infection, **the** tumor, **the** disease, **the** pain—"**It** is a problem that can be fixed." Thus, the ailment is not a part of your patient and his/her ability to resist. Rather it is something foreign and, therefore, considerably more capable of being influenced from outside suggestions.

"The pain might last a short while, and I'll give you medication for that, but I've seen it disappear in patients very much like yourself— often surprisingly fast. Don't be opposed to surprising yourself. You might wake up and FEEL 80% OR 60% OR EVEN 90% BETTER *[UNDERSCORING]. Call me tomorrow and let me know how well you do feel. And if you,* **John***, forget to take the pill…that's okay. Just know you can use it if* **the pain** *hasn't quite gone away yet."*

It is probably worth rereading that paragraph. Many caregivers, absent the Exquisite Art, would have delivered the message as follows:

"Your pain will probably last several days or more, so I'm prescribing you some pain medication. If it doesn't help, let me know and I can get you something stronger. Meantime, call me if your pain isn't gone within a week or two."

Suggestions offered by an Authority have an effect. This is the lesson of placebo. Therefore, the patient receiving the second of these messages will have been inadvertently cursed, probably by a well-meaning caregiver. And their pain will likely persist. Whereas the patient receiving the more Artful message will quite likely feel relief by tomorrow. This may be hard for you to believe in the absence of experience. But, as you move along the communication continuum, you will undoubtedly see what I have seen time and again. Patients, whether in response to waking suggestions or suggestions in trance, really can feel delightfully surprising comfort in all sorts of potentially painful situations, including childbirth, surgery, broken bones, injections, suturing, debridement and more. I urge you to begin using your new tools in these and other situations. And, as I often say: Don't be opposed to pleasantly surprising yourself.

Summing Up

We now have a well-founded appreciation for the power all caregivers wield as Authorities, and a deepening respect for the potential effects—positive or negative—of our words and gestures. We have learned when to use direct suggestion and when subtler approaches, like permissive language—including, indirection and metaphor—are more likely to evoke the desired response. Finally, we have combined the power of gestural UNDERSCORING with a subtle appreciation for the connotations of a few linguistic Pearls. It's a precious toolbox.

Now, let's begin to use these tools to build a grand edifice—the Exquisite Art of Caregiving.

"Language upon a silvered tongue affords enchantment enough."

—Salman Rushdie, *The Enchantress of Florence*

Chapter 5:

BLUEPRINTS FOR ARTFUL CAREGIVING

INFORMATION DELIVERY IS THE RECURRENT TASK of all caregivers. Yet, despite the fact that patients often hang on our every word, most caregivers rely on their good intentions and deliver those words haphazardly. It doesn't matter whether the message is a dietary recommendation, a treatment explanation, a diagnosis or a prognosis—casual talk is the norm.

What follows are examples of common patient/caregiver situations into which I have blended the various techniques we've been studying. In my experience, the results of this alchemy are often stunning. Not infrequently, I have watched "inevitable" side effects thwarted, panic allayed, pain averted, asthma relieved, renal colic eliminated. In time, I have no doubt your experiences will replicate and extend beyond these remarkable results. But remember, the following examples are drawn from long years of practice, trial and error. Be gentle on yourself as you begin. Mistakes and fumbles represent inevitable opportunities for learning and improving. If you heed Voltaire's admonition not to let the Best be the enemy of the Good, you will be richly rewarded. And so, too, will your patients.

Informed Consent

Let's begin with **Informed Consent**—an archetype for the many and varied situations in which caregivers find themselves having to explain an intervention, offer their reasoned opinion or disclose potential risks and benefits. In essence, Informed Consent as described below provides a blueprint for information delivery regarding any recommended treatment, procedure or course of action.

The Patient: A healthy 60-year-old man, Walter.

The Intervention: Routine colonoscopy.

The Benefits: Screening for colon cancer and premonitory lesions.

The Risks: Intestinal rupture, bleeding, infection, accidents of anesthesia, discomfort from the bowel preparation.

In this scenario, you will notice I use the various tools we acquired in the last chapter, including UNDERSCORING with eye contact and subtle voice strengthening (indicated by ALL CAPS). I also introduce a versatile set of hand maneuvers. Specifically, when discussing risks with the patient, I say: "On the one hand…" and extend my right hand, palm up, out and away from the patient. For example: "On the one hand," my right hand extending out and away, "there are rare risks that **some people might** experience." Those risks have thus been assigned, as it were, to a place out there away from the patient. Whereas, when discussing benefits, I say: "On the other hand…" and extend my left hand, palm up, and toward the patient. Hence: "On the other hand," my left hand extending toward the patient, "there are many patients, perhaps very much like YOU, who EXPERIENCE A COMFORTABLE AND SAFE EXAMINATION." This might seem a bit complicated when first read, but once you have practiced it a time or two it becomes easy and automatic.

Now, let's see how this technique, plus our previous learnings, all come together.

"Well, Walter, I'm happy to tell you your physical examination and lab tests are all normal."

"Wonderful. So…I guess that's it."

"It is, and yet there is one preventative measure I would like to encourage you to do."

"What's that, Doc?"

"It's a colonoscopy, which is when a specialist takes a direct look at the inside of the colon to be sure the tissue is all normal and that there are no suspicious lesions that **might** increase **someone's** risk of cancer."

"But I've heard that the procedure is dangerous."

"Well, let's consider the risks and benefits, shall we?" (For brevity here, I'll forego discussion of the bowel prep.)

"Please."

"As you may know, Walter, on the one hand [**right hand extends out and away**] everything we do in medicine has some risks, however rare; while on the other hand [**left hand extends toward Walter**] there are definitely benefits. Let's talk about the benefits first."

"Okay."

"The benefit of a colonoscopy [**left hand extends toward Walter**] is that, after cleaning out the bowels the night before, the specialist can directly visualize the colon to be sure it is healthy. To do this, light anesthesia is used so YOU CAN BE JUST COMFORTABLE [remember, ALL CAPS indicates underscoring with eyes and voice], and the scope is passed gently through the anus and into the colon."

"And what if he sees something unhealthy?"

"So if anything suspicious is observed, the doctor can either remove it—for example, if it's a polyp—or biopsy it, which means take a small piece for microscopic analysis, to be sure it's normal, healthy tissue. Patients DON'T NEED TO FEEL this, because of the anesthesia. And provided they have not taken any medicines [list them] that interfere with clotting, they can KEEP YOUR BLOOD where it belongs—NO BLEEDING. [That syntactic violation—from 'their blood,' which would have been syntactically correct, to 'YOUR BLOOD,' is intentional.] Thus, any potential problem can be spotted early and addressed."

Let's pause for a moment. So far, with very little extra effort we have:

1. Subtly assigned the risks elsewhere and the benefits to Walter (using hand gestures).
2. Avoided common curses like: "So we can see if **you have cancer…**" and instead, said: "…to be sure it is healthy." We have also avoided: "**You** might feel some pain or possibly **you** could bleed," by assigning those potential risks, instead, to "patients" and "they."
3. Inserted suggestions, using UNDERSCORING, for comfort, analgesia and hemostasis.

We know from placebo-controlled trials that our Authority can drive these suggestions to actualize in some 25–35% of patients. But the subtlety of our technique allows us to elude resistance and thus renders the likelihood of positive outcomes, presumably, even greater.

Now, let's continue.

*"I mentioned there were risks, so before I explain those let me emphasize that the vast majority of patients, WALTER, HAVE AN ABSOLUTELY UNCOMPLICATED PROCEDURE. Now, as I said, on the one hand [right hand extending away from Walter], there are **some patients** who **may** have complications, which **can** include discomfort, infection, bleeding or even, in very rare cases, rupture of the colon. Again, these are rare but **can** occur.*

"On the other hand, as we discussed [left hand directed toward patient],
WALTER, THERE ARE BENEFITS. *And since, in my view,*
the benefits outweigh the risks I am recommending you do this. I am
confident YOU WILL HAVE A SMOOTH AND EASY PROCEDURE.*"*

Note how permissive language ("can" or "may") subtly allows for the opposite possibilities (e.g., "cannot or may not") and so reduces the disquieting impact of disclosing potential complications—complications that are designated "out there," by virtue of our hand gestures and verbal references to **"some patients."** It boils down to this: Over there are **some patients** and certain complications that can occur; whereas, over here is Walter and a "SMOOTH AND EASY PROCEDURE" which can BE COMFORTABLE and during which he can KEEP YOUR OWN BLOOD.

People often ask, Is this honest? Is this fair? To understand the answer, we need to realize what goes on every day in traditional caregiving. Words and gestures affect outcomes whether we use them deliberately or haphazardly. The common practice of haphazard speech often leaves patients fearful and cursed with negative suggestions that can adversely influence their ultimate outcome: "**you** could bleed, **you** could experience a rupture of the colon… but whenever this happens, we have ways of addressing it, so you should be alright." Negative messages like this are commonplace.

So long as we honestly convey the necessary information, I would argue that only good can come from assigning the risks to "some people" and the potential benefits to our patients. Isn't that what you would want as a patient?

Returning to our exercise: If you imagine common situations in your own caregiving, and then rehearse the application of these gestural and verbal skills to those situations, mastery and unconscious fluidity will quickly ensue, as will the profound gratification that comes from doing it right and watching your patients benefit.

Defining the Symptom

When the drug Imitrex™ (sumatriptan) was first introduced for migraine treatment, I was excited to use it in the ED. However, I quickly discovered that while it was remarkably effective in alleviating headaches, Imitrex had one frequent and unfortunate side effect—transient chest pain and tightness. Often, this side effect would manifest 5 or 10 minutes after the injection, when no caregiver was at the patient's bedside. Despite forewarning patients, they were often fearful when, left alone in their room, they began to experience symptoms similar to a heart attack.

By then I had learned, as part of the Hypnotic Method, to "utilize" whatever stimuli the patient happens to be noticing. For example, if an entranced patient appears distracted by the slamming of a door, I would say something like: "And the sound of one door closing can be a pleasant indication of other deeper doors opening." Fortunately, the exigencies of the Emergency Department had also taught me that the same "utilization technique" also works for waking suggestion.

So, I decided that next time I administered Imitrex, I would "utilize" the scary side effect and connect it to a positive clinical outcome.

> *"This new medication called Imitrex is often highly effective and many patients, like* YOU, EXPERIENCE RAPID RELIEF *[UNDERSCORING].*
> *Now, I've learned that if a patient is lucky enough to experience a* MOMENTARY *chest tightening or pressure, which sometimes occurs,* **you** *will have almost* CERTAIN RELIEF *as the chest symptom subsides. It's as if, when one symptom disappears, so too will the headache."*

> *At this point, I would often have to leave the room, and the nurse would administer the injection. When I returned, 20 or 30 minutes later, here is what patients commonly reported:*

> *"So, how do you feel?" I would ask.*

"Lucky! It was just like you said. Nothing for a couple minutes. Then, I started to feel a bit of chest tightness, and I knew relief was on the way. I never thought I'd be so happy to have a little chest pain. But sure enough, as it disappeared so did my headache. Thanks, Doc. That's a great medicine."

Of course, many treatments have transient side effects: some are truly adverse, but many are relatively neutral. Left undefined, patients will often react to those neutral side effects with anxiety or dizziness, or some other vague and fearful symptoms. The Artful Caregiver proactively defines the side effect as a harbinger of therapeutic success. As the Imitrex example shows, this is especially useful when the side effects are known to be transitory and benign.

Here is one more example:

Knowing that the intravenous administration of morphine is often associated with a benign "head rush," I would routinely offer patients the following suggestion as I slowly administered the drug:

"Now, if you feel a slight 'head rush' coming on, you can take comfort in knowing this is the first sign that…REAL RELIEF IS ON THE WAY."

With this, patients would no longer complain of dizziness or even nausea, but rather greet the "head rush" with a gentle smile and the ready expectation of comfort.

The Practice of Letting Go

A wise old man once said, "If you can have a piece of an experience, you can have it all." I love this suggestion, and as you'll see, I use it to "seed" the idea that a tiny change here can lead to a large change everywhere. I will demonstrate this with asthma; but you can easily imagine this technique being used to elicit improvements in a wide range of conditions, such as arthritis, migraines, hypertension, dermatitis, etc.

The patient, a man in his mid-20s with a history of chronic asthma, has labored breathing and audible wheezing. He is cyanotic around the lips. The triage nurse has administered oxygen and called for the respiratory technician to provide inhaled beta-agonists. After introducing myself and obtaining a brief history, I move around to the gentleman's back to listen to his breath sounds.

"I see you're having a hard time breathing," I say, "so as I listen, it may help you to know that in medicine we think of the lungs as having four quadrants, two upper and two lower."

"Uh-huh."

"And I need to listen to each quadrant by itself...so, this is very important." At this point I place my stethoscope on his back, beginning in the right upper quadrant. "So, let me ask you to open your mouth and breathe hard in and out, focusing *just* on this right upper quadrant."

I would listen intently to the breath sounds, then say:

"That's it. Really hard breathing, wheezing *just here*. Good. Now, let this part relax...*really* relax...that's right, **even** more [OBSERVE >> RATIFY >> AUGMENT]. Remember, if you can have a piece of an experience...YOU CAN HAVE IT ALL. Now, let's focus over here."

I now listen to the left upper quadrant.

"Hard breathing now. Good. Really let me hear that wheezing *just here*. Good. Okay, now let this quadrant relax too...**even** more...that's right. **Really relax it.** And now let's focus on the lower quadrants."

I then repeat the exercise in the right and left lower quadrants, saying in the end:

*"Okay, now you can have it all—**just** relax all four quadrants and breathe easily." Removing my stethoscope, "I could hear you were really having to work hard, weren't you?" [Putting the hard work of breathing in the past.]*

"Yeah," he'd sigh.

"Well, your lungs have a way of letting us know. Rest easy now. We got the message; more relief is on the way. Meantime, I can see the oxygen is really helping YOU BREATHE EASY *already, isn't it?"*

> NOTE: Remember when we learned that avoiding mandates prevents resistance? Well, this last sentence is a mandate in disguise. The little tag-question "isn't it?" at the end is the disguise. Watch for these tag-questions as we move ahead; they are an exceedingly useful way of embedding commands without provoking resistance.

Many people mistakenly call this technique "Prescribing the Symptom." But let's look a bit more closely at what is really going on. First, whenever I suggest the patient exhibit the symptom, I circumscribe it: "Just here." Which implies, "…and nowhere else." Then, before moving to the next site, I instruct the patient to let go: "Now relax…really relax…that's right…even more." Finally, I unite these discrete relaxations with a global suggestion: "Very good. Now, you can have it all. JUST allow all four quadrants to REALLY RELAX AND LET GO."

Therapeutic Metaphors

We have already discussed metaphor as a method of Indirection. Now, I would like to discuss metaphor in the broader context of healing. In this application, we use our knowledge of the cause of a patient's illness to construct a story that directs the cure. Of course, all of our linguistic tools can be used in the telling of the tale.

For now, I will cite just two examples—one from the world of so-called organic illness, the other an undiagnosable syndrome (i.e., pelvic pain, etiology unknown). I have hundreds more. Many occurred during my days as an Emergency Physician; but many more have happened during the course of my daily life.

Skeptics will read these anecdotes and dismiss them with haughty pronouncements about the methods of science. They have a point. It is, indeed, time for noetic scientists to step up and elaborate a broader scientific basis for Noetic Medicine. But all science begins with description and proceeds gradually toward experimentation and precision. These anecdotes describe phenomena none of us were taught and very few think possible; yet, I witness cases like these nearly every week. Appendix II proposes a program of controlled clinical trials designed to place Noetic Medicine on firmer scientific soil. In the meantime, I invite you to consider the following technique (with minor variations) for relief of pain from gallstones, childbirth, coronary artery spasm, etc.

> *Jack, our handyman, is working in the backyard. On returning home, I saunter back to see how he is doing. His pallor strikes me at once.*
>
> *"Jack, you okay?"*
>
> *"Hi Doc, actually no. They say I have a kidney stone and it's stuck most of the way down, but can't get into the bladder. I'm not sure what that means, but it's been hurting for four days, and drinking lots of water isn't helping."*
>
> *"I can see it isn't. How 'bout if I explain what's going on inside. Getting a clearer understanding might help* YOU GET SOME RELIEF.*"*
>
> NOTE: I'm seeding the idea of RELIEF, using UNDERSCORING.
>
> *"Sure."*
>
> *"So, imagine the 'stone' isn't really a stone, but more like a tiny grain of sand—"*
>
> *"Yeah, they said it was only 3 millimeters."*

"Right. Now that grain of sand is trying to drop through the ureter, which you can imagine looks pretty much like a drinking straw." I depict the straw by holding my thumb and forefinger about a half-centimeter apart and moving from high to low, top to bottom.

"Okay."

"Only, at the bottom of the straw, there is this spasm which prevents the grain from dropping through." Now, at the imaginary bottom of the straw, I've formed a tight fist—signifying the spasm. Holding that fist, I now begin to subtly move it up and down in sync with Jack's breathing. My fist is held in front of me midway between the two of us, moving up as he inhales and down as he exhales.

"I see," says Jack, watching my fist.

"Now, what's nice to know is that for YOU to, JACK FEEL RELIEF all that really needs to happen is for that spasm to—" I move the fist up as Jack inhales, "LET GO and really RELAX." This last sentence is issued as Jack exhales, as he lets go, and along with the suggestion my fist relaxes completely so that my open hand now extends toward Jack.

"Uh-huh…"

"It doesn't need to happen this second, but when IT DOES HAPPEN, JACK, the little grain drops straight through and YOU FEEL NORMAL AGAIN."

Jack nods, then packs up and heads home. An hour later he calls my wife: "What's the deal with that husband of yours?" he asks.

"What do you mean?"

"Well, he did something to me. I don't know…he was just talking. But no sooner did I leave your place then this kidney stone pain I've been having…I don't know…it just disappeared. What did he do?"

See how it all comes together so beautifully? Permissive language, underscoring, metaphor (the fist)—and synching up with Jack's breathing (much more on this later). Think of it. For four long days this poor man suffered in ashen pain. Then, a couple minutes of seemingly casual talk, the simple sight of a fist relaxing and letting go, and…relief. Such is the magic of the therapeutic metaphor.

This next example occurred during a seminar I was teaching, while writing this book.

> *She is a new mother, her child only seven months old. In order to attend the seminar, she had to leave her baby with the father and drive several hours to the city. Now, at the end of the second day, she has a question.*
>
> *"I have a health problem," she tells me and the course coordinator, "and I have a feeling, based on what was discussed today, that you might be able to help. Can I have a few minutes of your time?" That day, we had discussed noetic causes of illness.*
>
> *"Sure," I say. "Can you tell me about the problem?" The young mother describes having had an IUD (intrauterine device) placed over three months ago. Initially, all went well. Then, about three or four weeks ago, she began to experience excruciating pelvic pain, without fever or discharge. The week before the seminar, she was hospitalized for three days. All the necessary tests—including ultrasound, MRI, cultures, labs, etc.—had been done. At length, the doctors could find no reason for her pain and discharged her with the diagnosis of pelvic pain, etiology unknown.*
>
> *"I know you won't know the answer to this question," I say, certain that because of the day's discussions she will know exactly what I am doing; "but if you had to guess…What do you think might be causing this now?" (A version of "Why today?")*
>
> *She pauses. "I don't know—"*

*"No, I know you don't know…but just guessing…**Why now?**" I press.*

Silence…and then: "I don't know…I mean, I suppose something to do with feeling guilty over leaving my baby."

There it is. Guilt. I will have much more to say, later, about guilt as a common contributory cause of human illness. For now, it serves our purposes to simply observe the role of metaphor in resolving this young mother's perplexing symptom.

"But you <u>know</u> you left your baby, right?"

"Yes…?"

*"And isn't **just knowing** often the worst punishment?"*

"Um…I'm not sure what you mean."

"Well, imagine a young girl or boy who does something wrong. What do you think they would rather have as punishment: a smart little smack on the wrist, and it is over; or, a year of scowling and criticism from their parent, who every day reminds them what they did wrong?"

A. This is a metaphor, in our sense of the word: a story about a child's punishment options.

B. Implied in this metaphor is that one punishment is worse than the other, and that suffering both punishments is NOT an option.

"The smart smack, and it is over," she replies.

"Exactly. People often forget that JUST KNOWING IS THE WORST PUNISHMENT. Of course, you'll always just know you temporarily left your little girl, won't you?" (The tag-question hides the command.)

"I suppose so. Yes. I'll never forget having to leave her." she says.

*"And so, you can **just know** that, even after THE PELVIC PAIN IS OVER. Can't you?"*

A. I am underscoring the embedded command, the ALL CAPS, using my eyes and voice.

B. She cannot "just know" (which means, "KNOW, and nothing else") while at the same time FEEL the pain. It is one or the other. And since she has already agreed that she will always know, she has to stop feeling.

"I suppose so." She answers.

"And can you imagine what a merciful God would say if He knew you had to forever-remember leaving your little girl, so you could come to a seminar to learn to be a better caregiver?"

"Um…"

"He would surely say: YOU'VE SUFFERED ENOUGH…YOU'VE SUFFERED ENOUGH. Right?"

"I suppose."

"I suppose, too. So, will you forgive me, I'm about out of time. I hope you won't be opposed to surprising yourself. Please, let me know how well you feel tomorrow." I am inducing her to forgive: first me and then, I hope, herself.

"Yes, of course. Thank you."

The next morning, this young mother reported to the course coordinator that she had awakened to discover her pelvic pain was gone. She had suffered for weeks, undergone an extensive and expensive workup, including hospitalization, and yet continued to suffer. Then, someone thought to ask, "Why now?" and to offer a therapeutic metaphor (and other well-crafted suggestions) directed at the newly revealed cause of her suffering.

This is how it all comes together. This is the Exquisite Art of Caregiving.

Summing Up

If words and gestures did not matter, if they did not affect outcomes, the techniques outlined above would be nothing more than verbal foppery. But the fact is, ideas evoke responses. And so, how ideas are expressed matters greatly.

When **Informed Consent** is delivered haphazardly, without care and attention, curses are inadvertently hurled like javelins at the very people caregivers are entrusted to protect. As a result, patients may depart their caregivers' offices fearful, dejected and alone—their outcomes biased negatively. Yet, done right Informed Consent can impart all the requisite information while instilling positive suggestions along with a sense of hope and alliance. Having learned to do it right, we as Artful Caregivers can now use the Informed Consent protocol to deliver information on virtually every kind of treatment or procedure.

Similarly, we can **Define the Symptom** whenever our patients are likely to experience some predictable, passing effect. Again, this method has broad utility, as a wide variety of treatments—herbal, manipulative, pharmacologic, etc.—elicit such predictable effects. Thus, for example, post-vaccination soreness can be defined as a prelude to a fortified immune system; or, a fleeting queasiness from some herbal remedy can be spoken of as the harbinger of rapid recovery.

The **Practice of Letting Go** embodies the elegance of Ericksonian healing, but without the trance. I find this method both speedy and versatile. I use it for a host of conditions, especially as they manifest acutely. "Show me what you've got, **just here** *[meaning, 'and nowhere else']*. That's right. Now, **let that go** and...."

Last, I will leave the myriad applications of **Therapeutic Metaphors** for you to explore and discover. This is an exercise that will enrich the rest of your career. Again, don't be opposed to surprising yourselves. I have no doubt your artful efforts will be wondrously rewarded.

PART II

Rethinking the Whole

So much for the Exquisite Art as it applies to various parts and pieces of a caregiver's work. In the next section, we will take a deep and thoughtful look at caregiving in its entirety—from start to finish, from complaint to cure. Our success will depend largely on understanding what health really is and how illness is caused. In this connection, it is interesting to note that traditional education does not address these topics explicitly. Instead, it is assumed we all know what health is. And, as to disease causation, it is implicit in the reductionist underpinnings of the science, but almost never discussed. The consequence of these omissions is often a haughty disdain for the inherent balance within the human organism and a peremptory dismissal of non-physical causes.

Having worked hard to refine our everyday communications, it is now time to refine our everyday thinking.

"All understanding, whether of the world or even of ourselves, depends on choosing the right metaphor. The metaphor we choose governs what we see."

—Iain Mcgilchrist, *The Master and His Emissary*

Chapter 6:
The Wisdom of the Body/Mind

THE WISDOM OF THE BODY is the title of a marvelous book, published in 1932, by the physiologist Walter Cannon. In it, he coined the term "homeostasis" to denote the body's dynamic capacity to maintain its internal equilibrium—in essence, the body's self-righting mechanisms. As in our discussion of consciousness, I find it useful when pondering Health and Illness to think of homeostasis metaphorically:

> *"It took generations to design the perfect gyroscope. This resplendent treasure can now withstand all manner of perturbation and retain its upright position. Strike its external frame with anything and it cannot be brought down. So long as the center spins, though it may tilt for a moment, a moment later the gyroscope returns to center. It is a marvelous thing."*

As I view it, the spinning center that powers and protects this gyroscope represents what is commonly referred to as "Host Defenses," the homeostatic mechanisms Dr. Cannon wrote of. Many components of that whirling core are now known: complex physiologic systems, the molecular details of humoral and cellular immunity, growth and necrosis factors, neural networks, etc. But many components of Host Defenses are yet to be discovered. I suspect that in the decades to come they will be spoken of in the language of information and energetics, and in other ways presently unfathomable. Known and unknown, the whirling activities of these components represent the evolved forces of survival.

> *"In a vacuum, the cyclonic center will swirl indefinitely. But exposed to the frictional forces of life—to injury, infection, toxic stress and noxious ideas—the gyroscope's center will weaken and slow. Usually, no one insult is sufficient. But over time multiple forces acting in concert will weary the thing, until at length a single blow from without can take it down."*

What is Health? Metaphorically, it is the gyro's capacity to recoil to center, to recover its dynamic balance. It is the ability to take the hits and remain standing—at times even, to be strengthened by the blows. Not that there will be no moments of distress, no off-kilter lapses—there will be. But the wisdom of the organism—the entire organism with its atoms and molecules, ideas and intentions—is to right itself.

What is Illness? Remaining with our metaphor, it is not the toppled top; nor is it the blow that brings it down, the final poke. Illness is the compromised core, the diminished Host Defenses—most often resulting not from a single opposing force, but from several. Notably, those forces can be self-imposed (e.g., a bad diet or unhealthy wishes) and/or they can come from without (e.g., microbes or negative suggestions).

Health and Homeostasis

The metaphor, however imperfect, illustrates two crucial points. First, rather than focus solely upon the presenting illness (i.e., the tilt of the gyro), we should instead enlarge our vision to include our patients' overall homeostatic capacities (i.e., the strength of the spin). We already do this to a limited extent with our routine physical assessments (e.g., blood samples, cardiograms, X-rays, etc.). But are we sufficiently comprehensive in our evaluations? Since we now know Mind Matters, in addition to assessing our patients' overall physical condition, shouldn't we also consider our patients' overall mental condition?

A surgeon friend recently told me that he learned long ago to postpone any operation toward which his patients felt foreboding. "Why so?" I asked. His response: "The only patient I ever had die on the table said before the surgery, 'Doc, I don't think I'm gonna make it through this one, but no matter what happens...thanks.'" The surgeon continued, "I only needed to hear that once." Somehow the patient had intuited a deep-seated "spin-impairment." Perhaps, it was an undetected physical factor—a blocked artery or an occult predisposition to arrhythmia. Or perhaps he sensed an unconscious noetic factor—an unhealthy wish. In the coming chapters, we will explore in depth how to discover and treat noetic factors affecting Host Defenses.

For now, it is important to understand that traditional allopathic interventions often target a single disruptive force—a microbe, a blockage, a tumor—and that while those interventions may succeed in diminishing or removing that force, they nonetheless depend on the body/mind's homeostatic mechanisms. For example, however perfect a surgery, it cannot succeed without the wondrous actions of the patient's healing systems. Absent those actions, the excision of a tumor would leave in its place but an oozing wound. As the remarkable surgeon Ambroise Pare observed four centuries ago, "I dressed his wounds, and God healed them." Likewise, however, perfect the psychiatric intervention, it cannot succeed without systems capable of learning, incorporating and growing. Returning to our metaphor: While our remedies may thwart an otherwise toppling blow, they nonetheless require a robust central spin to bring the gyro back to center. Neither can be ignored: not the offending blow, nor the whirling center. Our view of Health must comprehend both.

Therapeutic Restraint

The second point our metaphor illustrates is this: The human organism is an evolutionary treasure whose wisdom resides in its intricate and balanced homeostatic systems. Our first impulse, therefore, should always be toward Therapeutic Restraint: meaning, before undertaking any intervention—be it a simple leaf tea or a refined pharmaceutical, a hypnotic suggestion or a complex surgery—we should first consider whether to intervene at all. This applies to interventions both material and mental. Do the known benefits outweigh the certain risks? And beyond that, do the known benefits outweigh the uncertain risks—the unknown and unintended consequences of our ministrations?

Here a modicum of humility will serve us well, for the realm of "the unknown-known" (meaning, the knowledge that is out there, but of which we are unaware) is forever-widening. Take antibiotics, for example. We have all been taught that each time we prescribe an antibiotic, we contribute to selective pressures for resistant microorganisms. This is a "known-known" that rightly gives us pause. But most of us do not know all of a given drug's non-antibiotic effects. Tetracyclines, for example, are not only active against certain microorganisms; they also have proven effects on inflammation, proteolysis, angiogenesis, apoptosis, metal chelation, iontophoresis and bone metabolism. Most caregivers are utterly unaware of these "known" effects.

Even vitamins can have unintended and deleterious consequences. While caregivers of all stripes advise B-vitamins for patients with "low energy" and other non-specific conditions, how many of those caregivers know that B9 (folate) can accelerate the growth of certain solid tumors, even before they become clinically apparent? (*Nutr Rev.* 2009 Apr; 67(4): 206–212.)

And it is not only our physical interventions that entail uncertain risks and unintended consequences. What maturational milestones do we deprive our patients of when we intervene in their sorrows or meddle in their grief? Not that there aren't appropriate times and ways to step in. There are. But here, too, Therapeutic Restraint should guide us, lest our interventions deprive patients of the fortifying organicity of recovery. Most of us, for example, survived our first romantic break-up alone—though it was painful and disorienting. Yet, aren't we better for it? More certain of who we are and of what we can withstand in the future. Wasn't our central spin ultimately enhanced by the experience?

Summing Up

As caregivers, our primary responsibility is to preserve and strengthen our patients' dynamic capacity to maintain equilibrium. Health is that dynamic capacity. At times, this may entail discovering and dispelling the material and/or mental forces that beleaguer Host Defenses. At other times, it may require strengthening those defenses, through measured withholdings of treatment.

This is not to say Artful Caregivers should refrain altogether from offering treatments or remedies. Rather, it is to encourage caregivers to maintain a healthy skepticism—one that asks science and critical thinking to free our reluctant hands. As caregivers, we owe it to our patients to remain ever-mindful of the sacred wisdom and intricate balance that resides within all of us, a wisdom and balance we have only just begun to glimpse.

*"In this universe, humanity is like a foreigner just
arrived in a new city: we have grasped the basics of how
to get around, but there is still so much to learn."*

—Carlos Rovelli, *Anaximander*

Chapter 7:
THE NATURE OF SYMPTOM FORMATION

WE ARE AT AN IMPASSE. The traditional "Western" model of health and
healing teaches reductionist causes of illness, only. Tuberculosis, for example,
is caused by a bacterium. Kidney stones are caused by the crystallization of
solutes in urine. Heart attacks are caused by atherosclerotic plaques in coronary arteries. Each individual cause, so the teaching goes, refracts through
the lens of the body/mind to produce multiple signs and symptoms. Accordingly, a single blocked coronary artery may manifest as chest pain, shortness
of breath, tachycardia, anxiety, etc. But when one looks backward through
that refractive lens, all the various manifestations point to a single material cause—a blocked coronary artery. This method of analysis, peering back
through the refractive lens of the body/mind to identify a single material
cause, is known as "Ockham's razor." All Western physicians are taught to
think in this manner.

And yet, almost every patient I have treated with a heart attack, and asked,
"Why today?" has offered one or more plausible mental reasons for their
misfortune. Most often their answers have centered on romance, finance or
(perhaps surprisingly) moving, though there have been many other reasons
as well. How do these noetic "causes" comport with the standard reductionist model?

The simple answer is, they do not.

The Fallacy of Blunt Beginnings

Let me take an extreme example to illustrate the flaw in our traditional reasoning:

> *A despondent man sits at a private airfield where he once owned a plane, brooding over his plight. He is financially ruined, his wife has left him, he is about to become homeless. Some 30 feet away, another pilot fires up his single-engine Cessna. The despondent man can take it no more; he stands, turns toward the whirling propeller and walks into it.*
>
> *What caused this man's death?*
>
> *"The immediate cause of death was severe intracranial injury due to a rotating airplane propeller."*

I call this the **Fallacy of Blunt Beginnings**. Because the rotating propeller can explain all the identifiable physical injuries, it is designated "the beginning" of the causal sequence. All antecedent events, however necessary they might have been to the ultimate outcome, are ignored. Yet, there are clearly significant noetic factors that prompted the victim to walk into the rotating propeller: the dark wish to die being one of them. Are these not crucial factors in the causal sequence leading to this man's demise?

I suppose one could argue that all "beginnings" are arbitrary. As one Nobel prize-winning physicist once said: "I'm not so sure where you begin and I end." But even if designating a beginning is arbitrary, I would argue choosing the airplane propeller as the blunt beginning of this causal sequence is a poor choice, for it precludes insights that would enable us to better understand what really happened—insights that might help us predict and possibly prevent similar calamities in the future.

The same is true of the reductionist's blunt beginnings. In my experience, the etiology of many—if not most—human illnesses is multifactorial, with noetic factors often contributing. As we discussed in Chapter 2, ideas matter. So, why do our current causal notions of disease so stringently preclude noetic factors?

The answer is simple and telling. In order for science to make sense of Nature's dizzying complexity, researchers must isolate and restrict experimental conditions. This means scientists studying human health and healing often selectively ignore aspects of the whole organism in order to "control variables" and focus. Results from these "reduced" conditions are then extrapolated—usually, not by the laboratory scientists—to the whole organism, most often without regard to the emergent properties (e.g., physiologic systems, movements, mentation, etc.) that arise from the whole organism's layered complexity.

Reductionist Causal Modeling

Take warts, for example. Reductionist science has shown that human papillomavirus (HPV) infects immature skin cells and commandeers their intracellular machinery to form warts. Thus, the **Blunt Beginning** paradigm for warts is:

HPV >> CELLULAR INVASION >> INTRACELLULAR DISRUPTION >> WARTS

This is called a causal diagram. As we are about to see, using this simple modeling tool unlocks a whole new world of caregiving—one that comports with our most deeply held intuitions—and provides a framework for treatment, research and prediction extending far beyond the truncated model of the reductionists. As the brilliant Judea Pearl, in The Book of Why, has written: "Very often the structure of the diagram itself enables us to estimate all sorts of causal and counterfactual relationships: simple or complicated, deterministic or probabilistic, linear or nonlinear."

But first, let's acknowledge the achievements of the reductionist model. From it, we see plainly that the best way to avoid warts is to prevent HPV invading the cell in the first place. This observation has already resulted in successful vaccinations against many HPV strains. But what if the wart has already formed? Again, our rectilinear diagram proves fruitful, for it suggests that one must somehow reverse HPV's intracellular mischief—either by killing the virus upon entry or by disrupting its piratical capabilities. These are both worthy avenues for research that, again, are yielding useful treatments. So, there can be no doubting the practical value of the reductionist approach.

But how does the causal sequence above explain the following case history?

Gene's Story

He is a gynecological surgeon, and a gruff and surly one at that. "You might as well know at the outset—I think this is pure bullshit!" he declares upon entering my medical hypnosis office. "My wife sent me to see you, and I'm not happy about it."

"Nor am I," I assert, not because I feel that way, but rather to align my feelings with his as a Rapport maneuver. "In fact, the sooner we can succeed and have this over with, the happier I imagine we both will be."

"Exactly!" he says, plopping into the chair.

Gene (as I'll call him) is familiar to me, we are on staff at the same hospital. Not only is he known for his bitter temperament, but he is also a renowned penny-pincher. His wife has sent him to see me because he has literally hundreds of oozing warts over both hands, and the hospital is threatening to suspend his surgical privileges.

"Now, I hate to waste time and money," I say. "Don't you?"

"Can't stand it."

"And so, the fact that your wife has already scheduled four visits makes me think I am likely to be sitting here wasting my time when you no-show, especially since you have already called 'bullshit.'"

"Why should that bother you, I imagine she pre-paid?"

"She said you would pay," I answer. I then explain my fee, insisting he pay for the four visits in advance. I assure him if the cure comes sooner, I will refund his money.

He shells out the cash.

"And what if there's no cure at all?" he asks defiantly.

"It depends on our true goal," I counter. "If our goal is to fail, then we will have succeeded. However, if our goal is to be rid of those pesky warts, then we will have failed."

With that confusing comment, I had Gene's attention. The miser could make money back and succeed if he got rid of the warts fast; or, he could set his sights on failure and, by succeeding at that, waste money and time. The double bind is another useful tool in the Exquisite Art. We were off to a good start.

How Gene's warts disappeared was fascinating. They began disappearing after our first session, flattening and drying out. By the third session, the warts were gone—but not to Gene's eyes. Remarkably, he insisted they were unchanged, though his wife and I couldn't see them at all. We will never know with certainty why Gene "saw" them. Perhaps he unconsciously wanted to ensure the warts would never return, and so engineered a reason for all four sessions. Perhaps his ambivalence about working with me in the first place found expression in unconscious denial of what had plainly occurred. Who knows?

Whatever the reason, at our final session Gene, bellowed: "Whoa, are you ever lucky. I don't know how you did it, but those warts all seemed to drop off in the last two to three days. Look at this," he said, displaying his hands proudly. "Don't they look good?"

The treatment of warts using suggestive therapeutics has a long and well-documented history. In fact, as late as the 1990's the *Merck Manual* still listed "Hexing" (which involves therapeutic suggestion) among its recommended treatments for warts. In my long experience, I have not had a single patient with warts who did not respond well. Nevertheless, many caregivers question this approach and routinely resort to more painful and invasive measures. Why?

Remember our causal diagram:

HPV >> CELLULAR INVASION >> INTRACELLULAR DISRUPTION >> WARTS

As you can see, this model offers no explanation for what happened to Gene or to large numbers of other patients cured of their warts using therapeutic suggestion. There is no inlet for noetic causes; and so, they are peremptorily dismissed by physicians and other caregivers as irrelevant. Why bother to ask, "Why today?" if mental factors do not even feature in the causal sequence leading to the disease?

This is human nature, right? Most of us tend to doubt or disbelieve whatever lies beyond our received wisdom. In the late 19th century, for example, Newton's model of Gravity acting-at-a-distance was as sacrosanct as our reductionist science is today. Only a heretic would have dared to suggest that gravity might operate on a different principle. Well, a heretic and Sir Isaac himself:

> "That Gravity should be innate, inherent and essential to Matter,
> so that one Body may act upon another at a Distance thro' a Vacuum,
> without the Mediation of anything else…is to me so great an
> Absurdity, that I believe no Man who has in philosophical Matters
> a competent Faculty of thinking, can ever fall into it. Gravity
> must be caused by an Agent…but whether this Agent be material or
> immaterial, I have left to the Consideration of my Readers."

In this connection, we should recognize that, like Newton, the reductionist does not say of his/her discrete experiment: "This is it, this is the whole banana." It is not the tidy scientists who have misconstrued their own results, but rather the heady over-generalizers, who accept without caveat the notion that results from the petri dish tell the whole story: that cells in isolation experience the same influences as cells within a vibrant organism—which they do not. Those over-generalizers would do well to recall the old adage: absence of evidence is not evidence of absence. Meaning, in this case, not demonstrating the influence of noetic factors does not prove noetic factors play no role. Especially when we have good reason to believe they do.

Again, we are at an impasse. Or so it seems.

Expanded Causal Modeling

Fortunately, our perceived impasse creates an opportunity to expand our knowledge and capabilities. To requote from Thomas Kuhn's brilliant book, *The Structure of Scientific Revolutions*: "Discovery commences with the awareness of anomaly, i.e., with the recognition that nature has somehow violated the paradigm-induced expectations that govern normal science."

Gene's story is one such anomaly; there are thousands more. Therefore, we need to discover a way beyond the "paradigm-induced expectations" of reductionism. We need a more comprehensive model of disease causation—one that preserves the value of reductionist science but extends our understandings to include both material and mental causes. Ideally, this more comprehensive model will not only account for noetic causes of illness, but will also offer fresh insights into the nature of symptom formation and suggest new methods of prevention and treatment.

As you are about to see, that is exactly what the Expanded Causal Model accomplishes.

For some of you, the first time through this new model may be a bit laborious; but I assure you, grasping the implications of this new conception of disease causality will dispel much of the fog and fuzz inherent in our contemporary notions of health and healing. Moreover, once apprehended, the Expanded Causal Model will influence literally every facet of your patient/caregiver interactions, from history to treatment to cure.

Seven Zones of the Causal Diagram

Let's begin by dividing our new causal diagram into seven discrete zones, ranging from Zone I-Causes to Zone VII-Signs and Symptoms (Figure 1). We will examine each of these zones individually, as if they were static silos; but we should understand that this causal complex is really a dynamic welter of events in constant flux. Once we've examined the various elements of disease causation, we will then apply our new schema to Gene's case (and other cases, in later chapters) in order to gauge its overall utility.

Figure 1: Expanded Causal Diagram

Zones: I (Causes)	II	III	IV (Disease)	V	VI	VII (Signs and Symptoms)
Noetic Factors Mental						Organic: warts
Extrinsic Factors	HD	+PP	HPV Infection	-PP	HD	Social: withdrawal
Intrinsic Factors						Psychological: depression

HD = Host Defenses;　　+PP = Principle of Parsimony;　　-PP = Reverse Principle of Parsimony

Zone I-Causes

This zone includes all causal events impinging on the organism, regardless of mode (mental vs. physical/immanent vs. external). In this regard, the terms Noetic, Extrinsic, Intrinsic are organizing principles that allow for the convenient grouping of events; the boundaries of each category are non-critical. As Bertrand Russell observed: "…both mind and body are merely convenient ways of organizing events." Thus, "Noetic" refers to mental or psychological events like wishes and intentions; "Extrinsic" refers to external factors like diet, infectious agents and toxic exposures; and "Intrinsic" refers to internal factors like body temperature, blood pressure, endocrine and other bodily functions.

> NOTE: ALL ZONE I-CAUSES BOTH ACT ON, AND ARE ACTED UPON, BY ZONE II-HOST DEFENSES.

Zone II-Host Defenses

HD stands for Host Defenses (i.e, the central spin of our gyro). This includes all defenses: material and mental, known and unknown. I strongly suspect, based on the explosion of knowledge over the last 50 years, that science will continue to add to our understandings of these various agencies. Just think how little we knew about the immune system 50 years ago, and how much of its detailed complexity we currently understand. Who knows what new signals, cells and agencies are yet to be unveiled by the marvels of modern science? Meantime, we should understand that, taken all together, Host Defenses are what prevent physical and psychological perturbations from "toppling the top."

Zone III-Principle of Parsimony

This is the lens whereby as many causal factors as possible are answered/discharged/satisfied by the fewest number of diseases, ideally one: This is the **Principle of Parsimony,** the governing principle behind many, if not most, human illnesses. Thus, multiple Zone I-Causes press through Zone II-Host Defenses, eventuating (most often) in a single disease by virtue of this Zone III-Principle of Parsimony. Understanding this operative principle allows Artful Caregivers to grasp how it is that multiple causes so often find an economic answer in a single malady, and conversely, how treating those multiple causes is often necessary to prevent disease recurrence or so-called symptom substitution.

Zone IV-Disease

Disease is the single source (usually) that explains most, if not all, of the patient's varied manifestations. It is important to understand that as the Zone III-Principle of Parsimony operates, it "selects" from a multiplicity of potential disease options in a manner that satisfies the greatest number of Zone I-Causes. Thus, a disease will often have both material and mental causes—all contributing.

Zone V-Reverse Principle of Parsimony

This is the lens whereby the disease is refracted into its full range of possible manifestations, only some of which will penetrate Zone VI-Host Defenses to actually become signs and symptoms. This is the **Reverse Principle of Parsimony.** Looking backward through this lens gives us Ockham's razor—as noted earlier, one of the key diagnostic principles of traditional Western medicine.

Zone VI-Host Defenses

At this point in the causal sequence, Host Defenses effectively filter the Zone V array of possible manifestations, allowing only some of the disease's potential signs and symptoms through, while rebuffing others. Thus, owing to the strength of Zone VI-Host Defenses, a viral infection that could "refract" wildly into full-blown viremia and encephalopathy, is filtered down to, say, a few annoying cold symptoms.

Zone VII-Signs and Symptoms

Signs and Symptoms can be noetic and/or organic, mental and/or physical. The child who manufactures a cold so as to stay home from school, for example, may suffer from fever and tonsillar erythema while at the same time experiencing joy and relief from having avoided the threat that prompted his or her retreat into illness.

NOTE: Like Zone I-Causes, Zone VII-Signs and Symptoms both act on, and are acted upon, by Host Defenses.

The Expanded Causal Model in Practice

In practice, while I often think in terms of these seven zones and may even draw out a patient's Expanded Causal Diagram, I never speak of these various Zones or Principles with patients. That would be about as useful as explaining to a patient the details of the Krebs cycle or the workings of alcohol dehydrogenase. Rather, **I speak of ZONE II to ZONE VI as "the symptom-maker" or "the problem-solver"**—a functional agency within the unconscious body/

mind. Hence, there are "Causes" that press "the symptom-maker/problem-solver" for a solution. It, in turn, answers as many "Causes" as possible with a single solution—namely, one disease—manifesting as multiple "Signs and Symptoms." (Figure 2)

Figure 2: The Compressed Causal Diagram

Zone I (Causes) <> Zones II-VI (Symptom-maker/Problem-solver) <> Zone VII (Signs and Symptoms)

Gene's Story Revisited

In order to understand the power and reach this new paradigm offers caregivers, let's now reformulate Gene's case.

Gene had multiple Zone I-Causes. His history revealed that Gene drank alcohol somewhat immoderately, was a poor sleeper and was obese. Surely these "causes" pressed against Gene's Host Defenses, "slowing the gyro's spin." On the other hand, Host Defenses pressed back, maintaining a precarious equilibrium. For example, we can assume Gene's liver enzymes were induced, so as to deal with his alcohol intake; his sleep issues were countered, let us assume, by an adrenal response; and his obesity, though compromising, was likely compensated by cardiac and other mechanisms. In other words, his Zone II-Host Defenses were holding. Although the spin had slowed, it had not stopped.

Gene's emotions about his work-life crystallized into three forceful wishes, which added to the causal equation: (1) the wish to quit work; (2) the wish to draw disability insurance; and (3) the wish to maintain "the good life." Of course, there are Host Defenses (e.g., coping mechanisms) in the noetic realm, just as there are in the physical world. A strong noetic Host Defense might, for example, have countered all three wishes with one dominant directive—namely, the deeply entrenched resolve to repudiate "retreat into illness" ideas and to remain healthy at all times. We all know someone whose iron will is firmly set on staying well, and they do. But many people do not have such a deeply entrenched directive. In Gene's case, the absence of an ingrained "Only Healthy Solutions" principle, coupled with already diminished Host Defenses from physical causes, allowed the wishes to penetrated.

Three noetic causes now confront the Zone III-Principle of Parsimony (as do whatever other Zone I-Causes may also have gotten through, like HPV). There are always numerous potential solutions available for selection. For example, liver disease could be unleashed, due to Gene's alcohol consumption; or, a heart attack from some coronary vessel now silently compromised; or, perhaps, biliary colic from an undetected gallstone. The Principle of Parsimony operates to identify the one solution that best satisfies the greatest number of 'causes.' In this regard, the "gall stone option" is too transient to justify Gene's quitting work and drawing disability, whereas the other two options mentioned are too disabling to allow for "the good life." What about that latent HPV infection…couldn't that do the job by being allowed to run rampant over Gene's hands? The very hands he needs to perform his work.

Zone IV-Disease: The HPV Infection Is Activated.

Now, the Zone V-Reverse Principle of Parsimony splays out the potential manifestations of the infection, which include rampant skin lesions over the entire body, unchecked viremia, encephalopathy, self-contempt, shame, etc.

What prevents most of these *possible* symptoms from manifesting is the action of Zone VI-Host Defenses: these defenses, while somewhat diminished, allow Gene's hand warts to manifest along with some psychological symptoms, but at the same time they restrain all other potential manifestations. Remember, this is a dynamic balance: if the warts were to become infected, for example, they could exert backward pressure—weakening Host Defenses and thereby creating vulnerability to further spread and expression of the virus. Alternately, the very HDs that are now thwarting spread to the forearms and beyond could intensify and expel the warts from Gene's hands entirely. The end result is Gene's presenting syndrome: horrible hand warts, social withdrawal and depression.

In practice, we never work in this direction—from inciting causes to manifestations. Instead, the patient presents with an array of signs and symptoms, and we reason our way back through the Zone V-Reverse Principle of Parsimony lens—that is, using Ockham's razor. Of course, many caregivers stop when the Zone IV-Disease is discovered and resort to the bug-drug cookbook prescriptions of modern medicine. **The beauty of our new causal paradigm is that it tells us not to stop there, but rather to search (e.g., ask, "Why today?") for a multiplicity of contributing causes that, by working in concert, have weakened Host Defenses and ultimately found expression in the presenting syndrome. Those causes may be both physical and mental—organic and psychological.**

In this way, the new Expanded Causal Model almost writes the treatment plan itself:

I. Defuse as many contributory causal events as possible—mental and physical. Reducing the number of Zone I-Causes will result in both strengthening Host Defenses and diminishing the number of forces pressing for expression.

II. Strengthen Host Defenses directly, by all proven means—again, mental and physical. Here is where complementary measures (e.g., diet, exercise, self-help, psychotherapy and supplements, etc.) play a role.

III. Implement physical remedies, where indicated, along the reductionist pathway. Notice, the reductionist causal model has not been discarded; rather, it remains embedded in the Expanded Causal Diagram as Zones IV-VII.

We will return to these treatments in a moment.

But first, look what happens if we only pursue the reductionist remedy. The warts may fade, but the contributory causes and the diminished Host Defenses will likely persist. True, there are times when the disease's signs and symptoms are so discomfiting to the patient that he or she resolves to find a healthier approach: essentially reversing his/her unhealthful wishes and self-suggesting a cure. But this level of self-awareness and will power is relatively rare. More frequently, the initial Zone I-Causes persist. When this happens, either the treatment fails, or other illnesses soon crop up—so-called symptom substitution.

Now, back to Gene. Understand that Gene's "symptom-maker/problem-solver" had dealt him a fairly workable solution. Or so it seemed, initially. He could let the medical staff rescind his surgical privileges and, thereafter, claim disability insurance. But it turns out, Gene was conflicted. Part of him wanted the warts; part of him did not. Why?

> *"I've always taken pride in being hardworking, honest and high integrity. I'm not a sloucher." Gene says. "Getting kicked off staff and sent out to pasture just isn't really me."*
>
> *"What is you?" I ask.*
>
> *"I don't know."*
>
> *"What would you guess?"*
>
> *Silence. Then, after some time: "You know, I guess just retiring… not being a wussy and pretending some disability."*
>
> *"Because you are not a wussy, are you?" (Notice the tag-question disguising the suggestion.)*

In our sessions, I explained to Gene how "the symptom-maker/problem-solver" selects from a host of options in order to satisfy the pressing causes. When its reigning principle is "Only Health Solutions," illness is precluded and, perforce, healthy options are selected. I used hypnosis to associate that idea with Gene's self-conception: "…because that's what a hard-working, high integrity problem-solver should do…find Only Healthy Solutions…a healthy, honest retirement."

While in trance, I also offered suggestions like the following to strengthen Host Defenses:

"...and the body knows how to fend off viruses. We are all exposed to millions of them every day. And yet, you don't have a cold or flu now... and your arms and back and shoulders don't have the wart virus...and soon, your hands won't need to have them either."

Then, upon waking, I assign Gene a mantra to use during his time away from the office:

"Whenever you think of the warts, Gene, say the following 10 times. Mind you, it won't work if it is 9 times or 11. You need to say this 10 times: 'warts go away...warts go away...warts go away.'"

Having him focus on the 10 times adds a level of difficulty and forces Gene to focus and affirm to his "symptom-maker/problem-solver" that the current solution is unacceptable.

Ultimately, Gene retired with pride and dignity. He did not collect disability insurance; however, he did find other ways to support his lifestyle that were consonant with his self-conception. Meantime, his hands remained clear of warts, allowing him to play golf and "enjoy the good life." Two of Gene's three Zone I contributory noetic causes were thereby satisfied. The third, namely the wish to collect disability, was defused by (1) demonstrating how it conflicted with Gene's self-esteem, (2) fortifying Gene's Host Defenses through inculcation of the Authority-driven mantra "warts go away" and (3) inserting the "Only Healthy Solutions" proviso into Gene's Zone III Principle of Parsimony. Incidentally, Gene's Host Defenses were further strengthened through traditional counseling as to proper diet, exercise and alcohol consumption.

Of Causes and Cures

It is important to note that merely exposing contributory noetic factors, or nebulous emotions ("I hate work"), or ill-defined "stresses" does not generally result in a cure. This is a pervasive misconception. Catharsis is rarely curative; it only works when the patient has exceedingly strong ego function (a component of HD) and can successfully self-suggest: "That's not what I meant. Warts go away!" More commonly, the Authority of the Healer is needed as leverage to effectuate a cure.

Additionally, we should observe that while our new paradigm allows for noetic causes, it does not in any way diminish the influence of physical causes. Indeed, our Expanded Causal Model admits of all possible permutations. Some illnesses may be caused exclusively by noetic factors, whereas others may arise solely from physical causes. Regardless of the mix, success is always best assured by defusing as many Zone I-Causes as possible, while at the same time taking care to strengthen Host Defenses, amend the Principle of Parsimony ("Only Healthy Solutions") and interrupt reductionist causal sequences.

Summing Up

No longer are we constrained by the stunted and stultifying causal inferences of reductionist science. It is as if we have just been handed our passports and informed that the tiny town in which we live, despite earlier instruction, is not the whole world. Not even close. We are now free to explore the multiplicity of possible causes of disease antecedent to the blunt beginnings of the laboratory, to learn about the multifactorial nature of human illness, and to test the strengths and limitations of Noetic Medicine as it aims to defuse contributory noetic causes of human suffering.

It's time to put it all together—our expanded toolbox, our heightened reverence for the Wisdom of the Body and our expanded conception of disease causality. In the next chapter, we'll analyze the elements of the patient/caregiver encounter and begin to learn how the Exquisite Art restores wholeness to every aspect of our daily endeavors.

"Where causation is concerned, a grain of wise subjectivity tells us more about the real world than any amount of objectivity."

—Judea Pearl, *The Book of Why*

Chapter 8:
THE PATIENT/CAREGIVER RELATIONSHIP

ALL PATIENT/CAREGIVER ENCOUNTERS CONSIST, essentially, of three parts: (1) Information Gathering, (2) Synthesis and (3) Information Delivery. Traditional practitioners are taught to infuse each of these parts with the science and technology of their respective schools. We now need to add the nuances and understandings of the Exquisite Art to each part as well.

As you will see, our Expanded Causal Model dramatically influences what kind of information we seek, as well as how we synthesize a diagnosis and treatment plan. At the same time, our heightened awareness of the nature of statistical information and the Fallacy of Prophecy restrains and qualifies our prognostications, while Therapeutic Restraint gives us pause before prescribing. Perhaps most importantly, when the time for information delivery arrives, our new and improved communication skills help us to carefully craft our messages, to impart maximum benefit to our patients.

Let's begin by examining how this all plays out in the abstract. Then, we will focus on how one particular application of our reasoning saved the life of a man who conventional medicine, despite its many marvels, could not have saved.

Part I—Information Gathering

This first part of the patient/caregiver encounter includes the history, physical examination, laboratory tests, imaging studies and all other data relevant to the patient's complaint. What information to glean and how to acquire it are essential parts of our traditional education.

However, most Information Gathering is woefully incomplete. For example, the most important question in the patient's medical history (once the primary diagnosis is secured) is seldom asked, namely, "Why today?" Other important questions aimed at ferreting out common noetic factors are also routinely omitted. These factors often include unhealthy wishes, dangerous identifications, deep-seated guilt, etc. Moreover, questions aimed at determining what negative suggestions (i.e., curses) might now be operative are rarely, if ever, asked.

As you are about to see, the Expanded Causal Model redefines Information Gathering as the search for both the reductionist cause(s) of a given illness and the noetic factors potentially contributing to and sustaining that illness. Further, our new causal model provides a reasoned context in which to comprehensively explore the strengths or weaknesses of Host Defenses.

Part II—Synthesis

During Part II of the patient/caregiver encounter, the professional caregiver uses the information obtained in Part I to synthesize a diagnosis, treatment plan and prognosis. This entails the application of certain problem-solving principles, including anatomic and physiologic thinking, devising a differential diagnosis (a spectrum of possibilities), and systematically excluding diagnostic possibilities through the application of certain logical principles—including, as we've discussed, Ockham's razor—which seeks a single disease to explain the patient's presenting signs and symptoms.

As you might imagine, traditional Synthesis now requires an upgrade. The Expanded Causal Model reveals an etiology consisting of far more causes than the blunt beginning of traditional teachings; it also encourages, as noted above, a more comprehensive assessment of Host Defenses. Hence, once the diagnosis is secured, our treatment plan must now be targeted at both physical and psychological causes, as well as toward strengthening Host Defenses. As you will see in a moment, the good news is when the root causes of illness are extirpated, the prognosis for a lasting cure becomes far more favorable.

Part III: Information Delivery

As regards Parts I and II, we should understand that our patients expect us to be perfect. Not that we will be perfect, or even can be. But troubled as they are with their own fears and ailments, our patients remain unaware of their caregivers' personal strengths and weaknesses. They assume we have gathered the appropriate information and made perfect use of it.

They now hang on our every word. How we fashion and deliver those words will either help them or harm them. Here, our newly acquired toolbox will serve us and our patients well. As will our newly acquired understandings about the nature of health and healing.

Applying the Exquisite Art

Once again, science and traditional teaching must inform each part of the patient/caregiver encounter. However, the Exquisite Art can and should inhere in each element as well. For, absent the Art, traditional Information Gathering will fail to unearth key contributing causes of illness; absent the Art, the Synthesis will be based on incomplete models of causation and, possibly, fallacious reasoning; and absent the Art, Information Delivery will be haphazard and inadvertently deleterious. Most important, absent the Art, the opportunity to effectuate a real and lasting cure will often be missed.

This next case history illustrates, perhaps more than any other in my career, the vital importance of the Exquisite Art as applied to each and every segment of the patient/caregiver encounter.

Michael's Story

Michael is a 55-year-old Caucasian acupuncturist, a student of Chinese medicine and arts. While on a trip to China, he noticed a rubbery lump under his chin. Shortly after that, he noticed similar bumps in his groin. His sleep was disturbed by fever and night sweats.

After a "thorough history," physical exam, blood tests, imaging studies, and biopsy of the chin lesion, the doctors diagnosed lymphoma. Specifically, Michael had a rare and often-refractory form of lymphoma "caused by" a discrete genetic mutation.

Immediately upon securing the diagnosis, Michael started chemotherapy. He used his skills in Tai Chi and Asian arts to tolerate the side effects. It was tough. At first, the tumors shrank, and Michael felt buoyed and optimistic. Then, they returned in force: springing up like golf balls under his arms, in his groin and elsewhere.

The doctors tried multiple other chemotherapy regimens, all to no avail. As the tumors advanced, Michael's prospects grew dim.

Ultimately, a special chemo-agent was flown in from Germany. It was administered in brutally aggressive doses to annihilate the tumor long enough to allow Michael the opportunity for a bone marrow transplant. (His brother, it turned out, was a good match.) Initially, the transplant worked. Michaels's marrow was repopulated with his brother's cells, which began producing normal healthy cells.

Then, disaster struck. The grafted bone marrow cells began to identify Michael's body as foreign; they attacked, causing debilitating abdominal cramps, bloody diarrhea and jaundice. A virus (CMV), long-latent in his tissues, reactivated, adding insult to injury. Michael, who normally weighed 185lbs, quickly withered to 129lbs. Death was breathing down his neck.

At this juncture, science and traditional teachings had reached a fatal impasse. Chemicals had been used to kill cancer cells. Michael's brother's bone marrow had been transplanted to replace his own bone marrow. Other chemicals had been employed to kill pathogens and modulate adverse reactions. The whole magnificent machinery of reductionist science had been activated and deployed. Though countless others have been saved by these miraculous measures, Michael was not to be among them.

Just before graft versus host disease hit, Michael had been in the audience of a talk I was giving on the Nature of Symptom Formation. During that talk, I related a time in my Medical Hypnosis practice when five consecutive cases presented, each with guilt-engendered illness. For example, the first was a devoutly religious woman with disabling arthritis that began six months after the deaths of her two alcoholic sons. She blamed herself for their demise. The second was an equally devout woman with new-onset lupus, commencing five months after her bipolar father's violent suicide. She insisted she "should have done more," even though he left her the most beautiful father-to-daughter letter I have ever read. The third was a Catholic gentleman diagnosed with arthritis, who blamed himself for his son's substance abuse and was guilt-ridden over his own marital infidelity. And so on.

Shortly after that talk, Michael knocked on my door: "You know," he said, pale and exhausted, "something you said in that talk the other day, something about guilt…I just feel you can help me."

Here is what I learned in our first encounter.

I. Information Gathering

I took the usual history, as would any traditionally trained physician. Then, I began digging for causes and negative suggestions, "curses." If I had accepted that the sole cause of Michael's disease was a genetic mutation, I might have asked about family history and hazardous exposures, but little else. Instead, I began searching for noetic causes of the sort we've discussed in previous chapters—an unhealthy wish, an untoward identification, deep-seated guilt, etc.

Here is what I found. First, Michael—though a "devout non-theist" as an adult—was raised Catholic. He recalled, "the nuns teaching us guilt at an early age." (NOTE: The idea of guilt is often inculcated early in a child's upbringing. When hunting for occult causes, it does little good to know the patient's present faith. Better to ask about the faith and culture they were brought up in.)

Michael's father was a veteran who had suffered a traumatic brain injury during the war and was wheelchair-bound. "He was a patient most of his life." (NOTE: Most often, though not always, the young boy identifies with the father, the young girl with the mother. More than we care to acknowledge, this identification forms a driving current in the deep river of our lives.)

Michael's mother was a nurse who had cared for his father in the army field hospital. They had fallen in love, married and had four children. Michael was the third-born. (NOTE: Always look for the dominant themes—e.g., care, respect, dominance, disrespect, etc.—in the dynamics of the father/mother relationship.)

When Michael's dad was 54, he suffered a protracted seizure and died. Michael was 13 years old at the time. Upon receiving notice of his father's death, Michael did not cry. In fact, he admitted somewhat shamefully to having "felt a kind of relief." He explained that having a handicapped father had always made him "feel kinda different." (NOTE: Understand, this is a normal and common reaction for a young man in Michael's circumstances. Possessing this bit of wisdom allows you to reframe Michael's childhood impressions with adult understandings.)

His mother berated him for his coldness: "If you only knew how your father suffered!" (NOTE: The curse, discovered.)

A couple weeks after his father's death, Michael recalled spontaneously bursting into tears. "It hit me late, but hard."

Additionally, just before the onset of his symptoms, Michael had suffered a break up with his long-term girlfriend. He felt betrayed and angry. Yet, he desperately wanted her back. "I would have done anything to get her back." (NOTE: Hence, the admonition—be careful what you wish!)

In his misery, he had taken to "vaping" marijuana throughout the day, every day. (NOTE: A possible contributory exposure.)

Finally, when I asked Michael, "Why now?" when the mutation could have manifested a decade ago or a decade later, he said after the expected silence: "You know, I have no idea.... But I do find it interesting that this started at the same age as my father's death, 54. Maybe a genetic curse or something." (NOTE: Maybe, except the father did not die of lymphoma. Nevertheless, the answer strongly suggests that Michael's illness somehow relates back to the death of his father.)

The Lesson: When Information Gathering, hunt keenly for internal causes and external curses. Clearly, both exist in Michael's history. As we shall see, this is vital information and provides the key to Michael's cure.

II. Synthesis

Michael's primary diagnosis is established: Lymphoma *status post* allogeneic bone marrow transplant, with acute graft versus host disease and CMV infection. But is Michael's complex disease entirely the result of a single genetic mutation, or does his answer to "Why today?" hint at other contributory Zone 1-Causes that might themselves be amenable to treatment? To answer, we first need to understand a bit more about guilt, identification and the power of a wish.

Guilt

Pat, my assistant for many years, was born in Singapore and raised a Taoist. Late in her life, she married a wonderful man, a devout Southern Baptist, who asked her to join his church, which she did cheerfully. Pat enjoyed the hymns and sense of community. She flitted lightly over the dogma.

A year or so after joining, Pat said to me: "Dr. Steve, I have to ask you a question. I'm embarrassed to ask my husband or my preacher, because it's about something I feel I should already know."

You can ask me anything, I said.

"Okay," she said, her brow furrowing, "It's about guilt. I hear people talking about it in church and all…what is it? What do they mean, 'feel guilty'?"

My work had forced me to wrestle with this very question, so I was prepared. "Guilt," I explained, "has two components. The first is familiar to us all: it is that sense of shame or regret we feel when we know we've done something wrong."

Pat nodded passively.

"The second component is punishment," I said, "the punishment one feels they deserve for their wrongdoing. That punishment can come from the world, or it can come as divine retribution—from God."

For a moment, Pat's face was blank; then, her eyes glimmered: "Ha!" she exploded, slapping my shoulder and literally falling to the floor laughing. "Very funny, Dr. Steve…very funny!" Nonplussed, I just stood there. "Now," said my dear Taoist friend, "tell me what guilt really is."

I had done just that.

Everyone grieves differently; there is no right way. Michael's mother, drowning in her own grief, could not understand her young son's stolid reaction to his father's death. Almost reflexively, she cursed him for it, and he harbored the resultant guilt for decades: Something was wrong with him (shame), and he must be punished (retribution). What more suitable punishment than this: "Just wait until you are your father's age," rages the Avenger, "then you too shall suffer as he suffered—pain, debility and death!"

While much is inferred, my experience suggests guilt is likely a contributory cause of Michael's illness; especially since he affirms, "the nuns taught us guilt at an early age," and it was my lecture on guilt-engendered disease that brought him to my doorstep.

Identification

What Freud called the "imitative propensity" runs strong in all primates, including humans. Monkey see, monkey do. Perhaps Michael was so tightly identified with his father that his illness arose in response to an imitative imperative. Recall, the father had "been a patient" most of his life.

Identification is a potent and often neglected force in human health and behavior. I shall have much more to say on identification when we discuss *Rapport* in the chapter on hypnosis. For now, it is at least conceivable that an imitative imperative is somehow at play in the etiology of Michael's disease.

Wish Fulfillment

The wish: "to have her back, no matter what." The fulfillment: to retreat into illness, to become a patient and allow the strings of pity to draw her in. Michael had the perfect model for this in his childhood. His father had "been a patient" his whole life; his mother had remained the ever-faithful wife/nurse.

Perhaps, two powerful forces—identification with his patient/father AND the wish to have his girlfriend back "no matter what"—were conspiring, through the **Principle of Parsimony**, to make Michael ill and prevent his recovery.

> NOTE: In my experience, these "no matter what" wishes can be exceedingly powerful and often play a prominent role in disease causation. It is true, be careful what you wish. But, perhaps even

more important, be careful how you wish it. Better to specify the wish's precise form of fulfillment than to blindly consign its selection to one's unconscious agencies.

Understand, these possible noetic causes of Michael's illness (i.e., unconscious guilt, dangerous identification and an unhealthy wish) are not exclusive of material reductionist causes. Rather, they are in addition to such causes. As regards Michael's underlying genetics, for example, consider the following.

Genetics

Traditional reductionists might argue that a genetic mutation determined Michael's fate. Period. And yet, nowadays, a great number of scientists have been moved to concede that "Genetics is not Destiny." For 53 years, absent other contributory causes, the mutation did not penetrate Michael's life. It lay dormant, crouched and waiting. "Why today?" Isn't it entirely conceivable that other contributory ("epigenetic") causes were first necessary to weaken Michael's Host Defenses in order to allow the mutant gene to penetrate and find expression? And might not some of those causes have been noetic in nature?

Causal Inference

Let's construct an Expanded Causal Diagram based on what we have so far discovered and synthesized. Although Michael's cancer has been defeated for the time being, and he is currently dealing with downstream complications, a broad look at his initial predicament will likely prove fruitful. (Figure 3)

Figure 3: Michael's Expanded Causal Diagram

Zones: I (Causes)	II	III	IV	V	VI	VII (Signs and Symptoms)
Genetic Mutation						Lymph node enlargement
Guilt: Death wish			Cancer			Weakness, Weight loss
Wishes: "Retreat"	HD	PP	(GvHD)-PP		HD	Rash
Toxins: Vaping			(CMV)			Night sweats
Identification: Father						Fear, Shame, Withdrawal

Here we see multiple Zone I-Causes, all confronting, impairing and penetrating Zone II-Host Defenses (i.e., slowing the gyro's spin). Those factors are initially "answered" via the Principle of Parsimony with a single disease—i.e., cancer—which refracts through the Zone V-Reverse Principle of Parsimony and Zone VI-HDs to manifest as Michael's presenting syndrome.

His subsequent chemotherapy, then, further diminishes his already-compromised Host Defenses, even as Zone I noetic causes persist. Hence, even when the lymphoma is defeated, powerful factors continue to press for expression. The result is Graft versus Host Disease (GvHD), which further diminishes HD, and results in a recrudescence of CMV.

In other words, we have before us a dynamic and comprehensive causal model, one that includes both noetic and reductionist causes and effects, and that accounts not only for Michael's original disease (cancer) but also for his subsequent maladies (GvHD, CMV).

How does this more comprehensive view of causes and effects conduce to an effective treatment plan and prognosis—and ultimately save Michael's life? Let me break it down, step-by-step.

Diagnosis

Let's begin with what we can be certain of, followed by our reasoned suspicions.

What We Know

First, we know that Michael had lymphoma as a result, at least in part, of a genetic mutation. The lymphoma has been vanquished. However, Michael is now near death due to a vicious graft versus host disease and opportunistic infection.

What We Suspect

1. We suspect the punishment side of Michael's latent guilt revived on cue during his 54th year, prompting his "pre-ordained" suffering and imminent death. Now, at last, he will know the suffering his father endured.

2. Michael's imitative propensity—i.e., identification with his patient/father—might also be contributing to his decline.

3. Michael's wish to "have her back, no matter what" may have prompted a Retreat into Illness, in hopes of resuscitating the "I am a patient, she is caretaker" childhood paradigm.

Any or all of these factors could be operative to varying and unknowable degrees. We can never know which, if any, is most contributory to Michael's illness. Perhaps only one, perhaps all, perhaps none. Regardless, absent a successful intervention, Michael will be dead in days. He now weighs 129lbs.

So, why not address them all?

Treatment Plan

The treatment plan flows from the Expanded Causal Model. Observe how our approach now differs from the conventional/reductionist approach. Instead of thinking of Michael's various signs and symptoms as being caused by one disease, which arose as a result of a purely physical cause (i.e., the mutation), the Expanded Causal Model enables us to understand his illness as a consequence of persisting Zone I-Causes and diminished Host Defenses.

Unless or until those causes are defeated, the reductionist treatment of one ailment (say, cancer) will commonly eventuate in another ailment (say, GvHD) and then, another (CMV), and so on: **"endless endings,"** in which disease is but a hydra's head—the only true way to kill it being to strike at its heart—its root causes.

Our treatment must now be directed at those multiple causes, known and suspected. Additionally, general measures to enhance Host Defenses are no longer nice-to-have afterthoughts, but rather vital components of Michael's essential treatment protocol.

Let's look at how this lays out.

1. Continue Conventional Therapy (as long as needed)

This is an important precept in the Exquisite Art of Caregiving. Countless lives have been and will be saved by the traditional Western approach, which is aimed at interrupting a common causal pathway (e.g, mutation>>cancer >>symptoms), regardless of the antecedent factors. In essence, it is a "dam the river at its confluence, and you need not dam its tributaries" strategy.

In Michael's present predicament, combatting graft versus host disease with traditional measures might help contribute to restoring Host Defenses, which in turn might allow for suppression of the CMV infection. So, again: continue conventional therapy.

2. Target Deleterious Contributory Causes

In this case, we should presume that Michael's unconscious guilt, unhealthy wishes and dangerous identification are all Zone I contributory causes. Therefore, each of these causes needs to be addressed.

I will elaborate in later chapters precisely how to accomplish each of the following measures. For now, understand there are simple protocols for handling each of these common noetic causes of illness. Hence:

    A.   Defuse the "guilt bomb"
    B.   Sever dangerous identifications

C.   Nullify unhealthy wishes: e.g., retreat into illness

D.   Address unknown causes

3. Strengthen Host Defenses

I have witnessed accelerated wound healing in response to presurgical suggestions for "really rapid wound healing" in scores of patients. Think about what this means. All the healing agencies, which are a part of Host Defenses, respond to a single idea ("really rapid wound healing") and somehow collaborate to accelerate the processes of mending organs, connective tissue and integument. It's marvelous. Again, all in response to a simple therapeutic suggestion.

So why not offer similar suggestions in all applicable cases? "Really rapid healing." As was the case above, there are simple protocols for this, which I will elaborate in a later chapter. For now, let's include in our treatment plan: global suggestions for health and healing.

Additionally, strengthening Host Defenses should include scientifically proven advice as to proper nutrition, exercise, sleep and supplements. Let me emphasize "scientifically proven." Remember our discussion about the potential harm of folate supplementation in certain circumstances? In this regard, "natural" does not mean "safe," as I am sure Socrates would have said of his "all-natural" hemlock drink. Nor does "organic" mean harmless. Therefore, it is best to advise patients on what you know to be true and proven, while remaining skeptical of fads and folklore.

That said, it is fair to ask, what about placebo? Since it works in roughly 25–35% of cases, shouldn't we offer Michael some form of placebo? The short answer is: Yes, and we are doing just that. Remember, **inherent in every intervention is the Generic Placebo Suggestion**— "If you (X) undergo this procedure, then you will (Y) experience the prescribed outcome." Michael is presently receiving multiple medications that carry this implicit suggestion. Additionally, he is submitting to my various ministrations, which also carry an implicit placebo suggestion. So, concerning the inherent curative potential of placebo, Michael is covered.

NOTE: The time to administer an actual placebo—meaning an inert pill, procedure, injection, etc.—is when nothing else is being offered. This most often occurs when a patient is diagnosed with a transient viral syndrome. Just be certain that whatever you offer (e.g., a pill, an injection, a manipulation or treatment) is intrinsically neutral or beneficial and not harmful in any way.

4. Instill Hope and Alliance

This should be a part of every treatment plan, as hope and a sense of alliance with one's caregiver are what every patient wants and needs. Sometimes this is as simple as saying, "Miracles happen every day. Let's work together toward yours." In Michael's case, additional hope stems from the discovery that deleterious ideas are afoot, that they may be contributing to his illness and that those ideas can be defused or deactivated. While it is unlikely that I will elaborate on the specifics of those deleterious ideas directly to Michael, I can at least say: "Michael, based on what I've heard today, I am optimistic that we can work together and very shortly begin to see some remarkable results. Are you with me?"

We now have a diagnosis and treatment plan. The final formulation in this Synthesis is the prognosis. Often this is where the gravest mistakes are made. So, let's tread carefully.

Prognosis

Most people do not like uncertainty. But the future is always uncertain. When a patient asks, "What are my chances?" professional caregivers need to acknowledge that they really do not and cannot know. Further, caregivers should be ever-mindful of the fact that negative suggestions uttered by an Authority can have devastating consequences.

A frightened cancer patient asks: "How much time do I have, doctor?"

Before you answer, realize: Professional caregivers, all of us, live in a skewed world. When we are wrong, our patients rarely return to us. They go elsewhere. And if they do well elsewhere, they do not write to inform us of their success or our inaccuracy. On the other hand, when we are right, we cannot distinguish whether the predicted outcome is the result of our suggestions or of our material interventions. Therefore, we never really know whether our prognostic accuracy is the result of "the way things are" or the consequence of self-fulfilling suggestions. Remember how "a little pinch or bee sting" guaranteed a painful injection, whereas "an odd sound is coming, just listen" produced quite the opposite result? **Our experience is skewed toward prophesies fulfilled and outcomes predicted, while the wider world exhibits a far greater range of possibilities.**

Therefore, let's briefly revisit the two grand fallacies of prognostication that we discussed in Chapter 3.

The Fallacy of Prophecy

Perhaps without realizing it, many caregivers prognosticate simply to assuage their own fears and uncertainties. When a physician predicts a dire outcome, for example, "You have five months to live," he or she isn't so much eschewing "false hope" as espousing false certainty. They cannot possibly know their own tomorrow, much less their patient's. Besides, as I explained earlier, within that uncertainty resides hope. No matter what the ailment or condition, at least one person will defeat it and return to health. Perhaps the patient now seated before you is that person. Of course, this may or may not be true. But the pragmatic outflow of this conviction is that it will allow you and your patients to glimpse the unfailing flame of hope—however faint or frail.

Remember my patient, Althea?

Althea's Story

When I first met with Althea, I couldn't possibly have known that one day I would be sharing her story with medical students and physicians at the local university medical school, much less in a book intended for professional caregivers. "I have an 8-inch-wide pelvic lymphoma, biopsy-proven, and I think you can help me get rid of it." These were her first words.

The year was 1998. Althea was 33 years old and had an unremarkable past medical history. She had been thoroughly evaluated at Scripps Memorial Hospital, La Jolla, by physicians I know and respect. Several weeks before our meeting, she had undergone a biopsy. Her histologic diagnosis was "non-Hodgkin's lymphoma with moderate aplasia." Once the biopsy wounds were healed, she said, the doctors intended to commence chemotherapy.

The week before our meeting, Althea had encountered a renowned Indian Guru. He had lain hands on her and pronounced, "You will be cured." With that, she sought me out.

Our hypnosis sessions consisted of trance induction and deepening, with very few suggestions other than "only healthy cells." At the time, I had immersed myself in the work of Dr. Ainslie Meares, the great Australian physician-healer, and so Althea spent much of the session suspended, as it were, in "crystal clear stillness"—a place defined as "the zone wherein true and lasting healing occurs." Throughout, she remained buoyant and determined.

After six sessions, our time was up. Althea went for her pre-treatment MRI and then met with her oncologist to schedule chemotherapy. "Dr. Bierman, this is Dr. White."

We had known each other since our training days. "What have you done to my patient?" she inquired, her tone at once both sharp and a bit quizzical.

Unsure, I faltered, "Uh…what do you mean? Just some positive suggestions." Upon which her tone turned celebratory, "Althea's MRI shows the tumor is gone. Not a trace! I'm sending her for a PET scan to be sure…and presenting her to the tumor board next Tuesday."

It is now over 20 years and numerous PET scans since Dr. White's call. I have bumped into Althea at the store a time or two. Each time she assures me, "All's well. I'm completely healthy."

Think about it. A biopsy-proven non-Hodgkin's lymphoma with moderate aplasia, measuring 8 inches in diameter. Gone. The only intervention a few simple ideas offered by someone the patient perceived to be an Authority.

Anecdotes teach what is possible, and possibility ignites hope. No patient should ever have their hope extinguished. Therefore, remember Althea. Remember her as though she were your patient. Remember her, as I did, when an emaciated 129lb-man named Michael, with acute graft versus host disease shuffled into my office, pleading for help.

The Fallacy of Extrapolation

Again, statistics deal with groups, not individuals. Imagine, for example, that a study reports the chance of survival given a certain diagnosis and treatment is 1 out of 10. That conclusion derives from data on the study sample, not the general population or any other subgroup. If the study group is men only, be careful about extrapolating to women. If the study group is Caucasian Midwesterners, be careful about extrapolating to East Asians.

Even more important: Let's say the broad characteristics of the group match the broad characteristics (gender, race, occupation, weight, concurrent illness, etc.) of your patient. Still, beware extrapolating to your patient. Those broad characteristics do not necessarily determine individual outcomes. Your patient may have a unique confounding factor—a cellular or genetic variant, a supplement, an activity, a healer—that renders them far safer than anyone in the "matched" study group.

Moreover, "In a group of 100 <u>patients</u>, 10 of <u>them</u> will generally survive," offers no information about an individual's survival possibilities. The words "patients" and "them" refer generically to others; they are like blunt knobs that allow us to handle statistical information. As discussed, we mishandle that information when we assign it to a specific individual by using words like "you" and "your." For example, "**You** have two years to live," or "**Your** chances are 10%." Those words are more like daggers. Wielded by an Authority, they can penetrate and do harm.

This is not to say, never use specific referential indices: "Only after <u>you</u> are cured, will we know that <u>your</u> chances of survival were 100%." Just use them wisely.

So, what is Michael's prognosis? Studies show that for patients with Michael's constellation of signs and symptoms, mortality can range from 16–60% or higher. Do any of those patients know and practice Chi-Gung regularly? Do any of them have a competent medical hypnotherapist? On the other hand, how many of those patients went through as many debilitating rounds of chemotherapy as Michael? Bottom line: No one knows or can know.

"On the one hand (right hand extending away from the patient), we know that **some people** in this predicament are at serious risk of death. On the other hand (left hand extending toward Michael), we also know that patients, some perhaps very much like **YOU**, GO ON TO DEFEAT THIS THING AND LIVE A HEALTHY LIFE. Let's work together and hope that in retrospect we can see YOUR CHANCES OF RECOVERY ARE 100%."

And what if Michael asks, "But Doc, what are the odds? What do the studies show?"

"The studies show how patients in the selected groups behave. It is important for you to understand that those patients did not have your Chi-Gung skills, nor did they have a competent medical hypnotherapist at their side, nor do we know if they maintained your level of exercise and nutrition. That said, in some studies, up to 40% or more of those patients, MICHAEL, SURVIVE. (sic) And, if scientists were to select a group that perfectly matched your characteristics, I suspect YOU WILL SEE A MUCH HIGHER SURVIVAL RATE."

***

Part I-Information Gathering and Part II-Synthesis of the patient/caregiver encounter are now complete. We have gathered the information we need and synthesized a diagnosis, treatment plan and prognosis. Let's pause for a moment and ponder how very different these products are, now that we have stepped away from the microscope and viewed our patient in his or her entirety. It never was JUST the mutation. If it had been, the lymphoma could have developed decades ago. If it had been, defeating the lymphoma would have meant the end of Michael's woes. Instead, we see what commonly happens when Zone I-Causes persist: when one disease ends and another begins; when that one ends, and yet another begins…and another… and so on. Endless endings.

Our new Expanded Causal Model gives us hope. We have identified addressable causes, beyond the mere mutation. Our efforts to obliterate those causes begin now, with our first words and gestures, with Information Delivery.

III. Information Delivery

Michael has listened to my questions and answered them as thoroughly as possible. Up to now, all of my efforts and reasoning have been invisible and unknown to him. Yet, he expects (or, perhaps, now only hopes) that his information will be useful. Michael is more helpless and dependent than he has ever been. Death looms. His survival instincts are desperately seeking The One least uncertain. The Authority. And, like it or not, I am it. He now hangs on my every word, my every gesture. My reality is his reality.

Michael's Story Continued…

"So what do you think?" he asks hesitantly.

"You know, Michael, over the years, I've seen many patients, sitting like you in that very chair, EXPERIENCE MIRACULOUS RECOVERIES. The future is always a mystery. And yet, in considering your history, I'm confident there are issues we can address quickly. Resolving them can HAVE A PROFOUND EFFECT.
I've seen it before, as I say, in patients very much like yourself. Together, let's hope WE WILL SEE IT AGAIN." (Again, ALL CAPS indicates UNDERSCORING.)

"Well, that sounds promising. When...how do we start?"

"We may have started already...by just discussing the various influences that were there at the start of the illness. Let's agree on our goals first, and then, continue to move toward your cure."

There is a lot in an introduction like that. As we discussed earlier, confusion ("we may have started already") focuses attention; "various influences that **were** there" implies multiple causes, now in the past, and the deliberate UNDERSCORING embeds curative suggestions.

Michael and I agreed on the goal (more on this in the next chapter): "Health and engagement in life." I then implemented the following treatment plan, using both waking suggestion (as in the introductory talk above) and hypnotic trance:

A.   Continue conventional therapy as long as needed

B.   Target Deleterious Causes

- Defuse the "guilt bomb"
- Deal with the dangerous identification
- Nullify the retreat into illness and other unhealthy wishes
- Address unknown causes

C.   Strengthen Host Defenses

- Global suggestions for health and healing

I scheduled two hours for each session and expected Michael to do the same. In the first session, we spent slightly more than the allotted time. Subsequent sessions tended to be shorter. Total treatment time was approximately eight hours over four sessions. (Contrast this with the hundreds of hours already devoted to Michael's traditional medical treatments.)

After the very first session, Michael began to gain weight. "At that moment," he later recalled, "I felt a change. I was no longer a patient. I was me—a survivor."

Today, over 10 years later, Michael is still a survivor—happy, healthy and married to a wonderful woman. He now weighs 178lbs. Remember his goal? "Health and engagement in life."

The "how-to" details of treating Michael's noetic causes are important and will be the focus of Chapter 12. Before that, however, we need to acquire what many consider the ultimate refinement along the communication continuum—namely, the ability to induce and utilize hypnotic trance. While that may sound daunting to those unfamiliar with the Hypnotic Method, I can assure you it is simply a natural progression along the path you are already on.

Summing Up

Michael's case does not represent a "series of one," as some disdainful practitioners might wrongly assert. I have used this basic approach on cardiac patients with advanced disease who have undergone numerous invasive procedures and are on highly toxic drugs, only to see them weaned off their medications and returned to normal life. I have applied this method to Stage 4 cancer patients, who have swiftly "turned the corner" and gotten on with healthy living. And likewise, with patients suffering autoimmune diseases, psychotic depression, refractory pain syndromes and numerous other bodily afflictions.

Noetic causes can wear down Host Defenses and find expression in disease. This is a simple fact of human existence. This does not mean that noetic causes reside in the etiology of every disease; that is as unlikely as the proposition that physical causes underlie all human illnesses. But a failure to search for noetic causes, and to act on them when discovered—that is an error with potentially grave consequences, as Michael's case clearly attests. Fortunately, as we learned early on, the door swings both ways. If ideas can cause or contribute to disease, then other ideas can cause or contribute to healing.

The lesson here is to look for patients who manifest "endless endings." Ask those patients, "Why now?" or "Why today?" Then, wait…listen. Will it be an unhealthy wish, a dangerous identification, a retreat into illness? Will it be the residue of some adverse conditioning event? Be patient in your silence, and the answers will come.

Artful Applications and Exquisite Outcomes

The refinements in communication and thinking that we have studied in Parts I and II enhance a caregiver's power to influence healthful outcomes tremendously. No additional skills are needed for most patients or situations. However, there are times when circumstances are so dire or causes so deep, that every ounce of influence a caregiver can marshal is needed. A sliver of enhanced power may save a life.

In this next section, we will look at a further refinement along the communication continuum—hypnotic trance—and we will explore how and when to apply it safely and effectively. With a tool so powerful, it behooves us first to consider the ethics of its use. After that, we will proceed to the marvels of bloodless surgery and the stunning "deep cures" that come from treating common noetic causes of illness.

Of course, not all caregivers can find time to treat patients in the manner outlined below. Nor will they need to. As we will soon see, much of what can be learned from the Hypnotic Method is readily adaptable to the rush and hurry of daily practice. Moreover, it is my experience that once Artful Caregivers learn how to induce bloodless surgeries and address the root causes of illness, many begin to carve out time to practice those skills. Often, those times are among the most gratifying experiences of their careers.

"But we were often handicapped…, for we always found that the cerebral hemispheres were sensitive to far finer gradations of stimulus than we could furnish."

—I. P. Pavlov (1924)

Chapter 9:
ETHICS—A COMPASS FOR CAREGIVERS

MY FIRST PRESURGICAL HYPNOSIS PATIENT, as you may recall, was a lady named Jan. She had ulcerative colitis, and her inflamed colon had troubled her for decades. "I'm done with this colon," she announced. "I want it out."

By coincidence, the patient I had just finished treating, Brad, also had ulcerative colitis. When Brad presented, he was on high dose steroids and other toxic medications. We worked together for six sessions, and his response was remarkably positive. That was 24 years ago. Recently, I treated Brad's wife for a minor condition and learned that since our time together, Brad has never required steroid treatment and, with few exceptions, has remained asymptomatic throughout the years.

Naturally, I believed I could cure Jan, or at the very least, quell her inflammation sufficiently to allow her to keep her colon. "Nope, that's not what I want," she insisted, after hearing me out. "I just want a smooth surgery. I don't mind playing golf while wearing a bag (i.e., colostomy bag)." She was scheduled for a total colectomy the following week.

What do you do? Here is a perfectly competent adult who, despite your experience and advice to the contrary, has decided to have a vital organ removed and wear a bag for the rest of her life.

Perhaps the best way to answer this question is to consider what might have happened if, while treating Jan, I had insinuated suggestions for improvement of her underlying condition. Would those efforts have changed her mind about surgery? Probably not. Jan had already resolved to undergo the procedure. However, because I would have violated her trust and inserted subliminal suggestions contrary to her wishes, it is likely her defensive mechanisms—even while in trance—would have activated. Those defenses are blunt psychological tools: not forceps and scalpels, more like spades and hammers. Recognizing the invasion, Jan might have unconsciously bludgeoned my suggestions—not only those for symptom relief but also suggestions for hemostasis, wound healing and comfort.

> *As an old Taoist priest once told me: "Trust is a crystal rice bowl. Break it and no matter how hard you try, it will never be the same."*

I explained to Jan my prior success in treating her condition and offered to work toward the same outcome with her. It was a warm and honest discussion, but at length, she made her wishes clear. Based on those wishes, and those alone, we proceeded. Surprisingly (remember, this was my first such case), Jan lost almost no blood during surgery, woke and remained comfortable throughout her hospitalization and healed with stunning celerity. Had I violated her trust and inserted suggestions to quell the inflammation, I doubt we would have celebrated such a convincing success.

The Caregiver's Covenant

Clinical success is optimized when goals are shared, when caregivers and patients work together toward a common end. Of course, for two people to share a goal, they must first understand it and then agree to pursue it together. Sounds simple. And yet, misunderstandings over so-called shared goals are a commonplace. Take marriage, for example. When two people proclaim their love for each other and marry, it is assumed they share a common goal. After all, isn't that what "love" means? Later, a fair percentage of married couples discover that "love" can mean different things to different people. Likewise, with many business partnerships. Even in the realm of healing, these kinds of misunderstandings abound. In psychiatry, for example, a patient declares their wish to be "more confident" and then therapy proceeds toward that goal. But what really is that goal? How do you recognize it when you get there? What specifically will it feel like and look like? Isn't it fair to assume that "more confident" must have a wide variety of meanings?

My usual manner of defining a patient's goal looks for specific verifiable ways in which to recognize and understand it, before proceeding. Further, that goal needs to be stated in the positive. It is not adequate to say, "I want to be pain-free." As Artful Caregivers, we need to ask:

"And when you are pain-free, what will you be?"

"Comfortable, I suppose."

"Comfortable? Where, and while doing what?"

"From morning to night, bending and lifting."

"And what will your state of mind be when you are comfortable from morning to night, bending and lifting?"

"Grateful, I guess."

"And how might you experience that gratitude?"

"Smiling and breathing, open and full."

"So, is it fair to say: 'Our goal is for you to be comfortable—meaning, able to bend and lift with a smile on your face and easy breathing—morning to night?'"

"Yes, that is it exactly."

In the previous chapter, I wrote of Michael's stated goal as: "Healthy and engaged in life." As is, this is one of those fluffy nebulosities that can mean a thousand things. Rest assured, during our first session Michael and I spent considerable time defining specifically what the goal meant and how we would recognize it. For example, one component of "health" was "sustainably regaining 50–60lbs of muscle." "Engaged in life," denoted "having a loving relationship with someone special—a relationship filled with warmth and laughter and easy silences." Each component was explored down to what it will actually feel/look/sound like when achieved.

In other words, in defining a patient's goals, nothing should be left to your imagination. Both you and your patient should understand exactly what success looks and feels like, so that when it is achieved you can recognize and celebrate success together. Once the patient's goals are sharply defined in verifiable terms, those goals become your goals, and the potent tools we are about to explore become assets devoted solely to the achievement of those ends.

I call this the Caregiver's Covenant—an inviolable pact between patients and practitioners of the Exquisite Art.

Curative Intent

Humans communicate verbally and nonverbally. Accordingly, we have devoted considerable time to both verbal and gestural communication techniques in the Exquisite Art of Caregiving. What we have not discussed is something far subtler, namely, the effect of the caregiver's mind-set. The question is: Can a caregiver's unspoken suppositions about the patient's ultimate prospects exert an influence on that patient's outcome?

In recent years, an extensive discipline on nonverbal communication has emerged, demonstrating that telltale signs—e.g., subtle facial expressions, colorations, pupillary responses, micro-muscular movements, etc.—can often signal our underlying thoughts. As Bill Bryson points out in *The Body*, "...we all indulge in 'microexpressions'—flashes of emotion, no more than a quarter of a second in duration, that betray our true inner feelings regardless of what our more general, controlled expression is conveying." Patients detect those microexpressions and decode that information. And while their interpretations may or may not be accurate, the fact that this auxiliary channel of communication exists obliges us to be self-aware and cautious, especially in approaching patients toward whom we are negatively disposed or about whose outcomes we are pessimistic.

Consider:

> *My friend Jack is nearly dead. A recurrence of diffuse large B-cell lymphoma has infiltrated his brain and cranial nerves. His eye movements are dysconjugate, speech is slurred, mental status is… shaky at best.*
>
> *Outside his hospital door, the doctors are speaking and do not notice me: "We can keep him comfortable…Yes, it won't be long…Let's not get too aggressive here." They all believe he will die soon. None recalls the hopeful words of Dr. Bernie Siegel in* Love, Medicine & Miracles: *"Far better to admit that the situation is grave, yet to remind the patient in truth that there is no 'incurable' disease from which someone has not recovered, even at the threshold of death."*
>
> *Years earlier, I had done presurgical hypnosis on Jack for a double knee replacement. Four days after surgery he called me: "Steve, you gotta put me in your book. I want royalties."*
>
> *"What's going on, Jack," I asked.*
>
> *"Well, they're kicking me out of rehab today. Say I'm no good for morale. Gotta be honest, I guess I've been showin' off a bit." Turns out, on day four post-op., Jack was going up and down stairs and bragging about it, while others with similar surgeries were groaning through physical therapy. Owing to this success, my Authority with Jack in matters medical is substantial.*

While the doctors continue to talk outside, I move into Jack's room. I know it is life or death for my friend. "Jack," I say, with little finesse, "you've got a decision here and only you can make it." That gets his attention. "You remember when you bounded up the stairs after your knee surgery?" He chuckles. "You remember how your stitches healed faster than your surgeon had ever seen?"

He nods.

"You know YOUR UNCONSCIOUS IS A POWERFUL THING THAT CAN SURPRISE EVEN THE BEST DOCTORS, right?"

"Right," he mutters weakly.

"Well, Jack, now it's TIME FOR YOUR UNCONSCIOUS TO GO TO WORK again. KILL THE TUMOR and surprise all these doubting doctors." I tell Jack and his wife that I have overheard their pessimistic talk. "But they don't know you, Jack, and I do. You wanna live?"

"Sure do," he says.

"Then you tell these young doctors exactly that, because they need to know it. And then SHOW THEM WHAT THAT STUNNING SICILIAN IMMUNE SYSTEM OF YOURS IS CAPABLE OF. You hear me, Jack…it's miracle time. Let's go!"

When the doctors walk in minutes later, Jack hears them out. None of them gives voice to their pessimism; their despair is well-hidden. But once they have finished, as if possessed, Jack conjures his strongest voice and reads them the riot act: "I want nothing less than a cure," he insists. "A cure, I tell you. And if you are not ready to make that happen then you can all just leave. Because there is one thing you all need to know…I am walking out of this hospital under my own power. So, you're either with me or against me…and if you're against me… get out now!"

Imagine if I had not heard the doctors' mutterings and had not steeled my friend against their dark ideas. Despite the doctors' discretion, Jack might nonetheless have "decoded" the doctors' unspoken message, "Death is imminent." And had that happened, isn't it at least conceivable that harm would have been done?

Many would say Jack was "terminal." After all, the recurrence of his lymphoma in the central nervous system was ominous. His cranial nerves were infiltrated, his mentation was foggy, his eyes proptotic; he had wounds that would not heal and blood clots in his legs. But that day, that moment in the hospital, when I used my accrued Authority and the refinements of permissive language and UNDERSCORING to awaken his prodigious healing capacities—that moment turned the tide.

> *A year and a half later, while Jack was visiting a friend in the same hospital, he bumped into one of the oncology fellows who had treated him:*
>
> *"Mr. Sparacio! My God is that you—" blurted the ashen young doctor in disbelief. He had apparently rotated off service and presumed Jack was dead.*
>
> *"Damn right, it is," snapped Jack, savoring the moment.*
>
> *"I-I-I…" stammered the fellow.*
>
> *"Let that be a lesson to you, young man," said Jack triumphantly, as he turned and walked away.*

Let that be a lesson to all caregivers. It was for me.

Artful Caregivers serve their patients best by holding in their thoughts the possibility of a cure—no matter how dire the circumstances. **Miracles do happen and hope for a miracle is never false hope.**

What About Chronic Disease?

One of my dear colleagues once asked, "But what of type I diabetes mellitus? Is it wrong to tell a patient, 'There is no cure. You'll just have to learn to live with it'?" My answer is simple: It is wrong to even think that way—to believe there is no hope and convey that hopelessness to your patient.

Let me explain.

Caregivers need to understand that their belief a disease or condition is incurable is an act of faith, not of science. It is absurd to hide behind the mantle of science and claim knowledge of something you do not and cannot know. A seasoned endocrinologist might see 10,000 patients with Type I DM during his/her career. That's 10,000 out of the 1.25 million in the United States today. Do you think if one of those patients had experienced a spontaneous "remission," they would have returned to that endocrinologist to enlighten him? Certainly not, for they would have feared his begrudging curse: "Well, I'm happy for you. Enjoy it while you can…before it returns." Nor could such an endocrinologist possibly know everything that is going on in every research facility around the world—in China, Japan, India, Europe. And even if he or she did, a serendipitous finding in some unrelated field might very well yield an unexpected cure.

A better way to think about such diseases is to hold in your thoughts the words of Dr. Siegel, which bear repeating: "…there is no 'incurable' disease from which someone has not recovered, even at the threshold of death." While at times this, too, may seem a faith-based belief— remember my friend, Jack; remember Michael; remember Charlene; remember my mother-in-law Michele; remember Althea. These are not just stories; these are people. And these are not remissions, they are cures.

A better way to inform patients about this kind of diagnosis is as follows:

You: Good morning, Jason. I got your tests back, and they tell us this: We have some things to deal with today, and some things to hope for tomorrow.

Jason: Huh?

You: Well, on the one hand, the tests show you have diabetes, and so we will need to manage that with medicine and diet and some new habits to ensure, JASON YOU CONTINUE A NORMAL HEALTHY LIFE.

Jason: So, it is diabetes…damn.

You: Yes…but here is something really important for you to know about diabetes…that a lot of people might not understand: As a great physician once said, "There is no disease from which someone has not recovered fully." And that includes diabetes. So, no matter how rare the occurrence, and it is rare, THERE IS ALWAYS THAT CHANCE.

Jason: Really…that's nice to know.

You: Yes. And beyond that, just as medical science is advancing against cancer and infection…so, too, is it advancing against diabetes. Remember, miracles happen every day. Who knows what kind of cures will be discovered tomorrow? Or even what your own "physician within" may, JASON, DO IN THE WAY OF HEALING YOURSELF?

Jason: Yeah…I mean, I guess—

You: In the meantime, let's get to work, keeping you healthy. (Then, go on to your informed consent protocol as applied to insulin therapy, etc.)

Summing Up

There is, of course, an exception to the rule of Curative Intent. But it's not what many doctors believe it to be, especially those who deal with "chronic disease." Unfortunately, such doctors will often read "hope for a miracle is never false hope" as the slogan of some cheery, albeit naïve, optimist. It is not. The time to surrender your hope for a cure is not upon diagnosing a disease that is currently without remedy. As you will read shortly, by expanding our conception of disease causation, we gain access to new methods of effecting cures. Using those methods, for example, I have witnessed tumors disappear, autoimmune diseases resolve, refractory mental disorders (so-called fixed characterological disorders) abate and advanced heart disease relent—all as a result of treating deeply rooted noetic causes.

Moreover, the triumphs of modern medical science will surely continue to march on. As David Deutsch said: "...we really should understand all our predictions as implicitly including the proviso 'unless the creation of new knowledge intervenes.'" And new knowledge will intervene. The time, then, to abandon Curative Intent is not when our ignorance of the future, skewed vision of the present and emotional exhaustion from work all conspire to produce a defensive pessimism. Those dark forces must forever be battled back. The time to abandon Curative Intent is ONLY when our ailing patient (or their legal advocate) has clearly and competently decided, in the absence of a treatable or self-limited depression, that it is time to die. Then, and only then, do the skills and wisdoms of the Artful Caregiver bend toward a digni-fied and peaceful end.

Until that time comes, our patients' best outcomes will follow when shared goals and Curative Intent guide the healing efforts of their caregivers.

"I begin by saying to the patient that I believe benefit is to be derived from the use of suggestive therapeutics, that it is possible to cure or to relieve him..."

—H. Bernheim, M.D. (1884)

Chapter 10:

HYPNOSIS FOR EVERYDAY CAREGIVING

SO FAR, WE HAVE LARGELY EXPLORED WAYS to improve and empower our everyday practice by skillfully imparting salutary ideas in the usual course of events. We now have a communication toolbox and blue-prints for action that will yield stunning results, especially when exercised artfully on patients who trust our Authority.

But what healthful influence can we exert when we have little, if any, Authority? How can we help when the situation is perilous, but the patient is a family member or friend, well-aware of our foibles and fallibilities, or when the patient is a stranger, who knows little if anything about us, or a cynic, who trusts virtually no one?

Consider, for example, a presurgical patient. Unless you are the surgeon or anesthesiologist, your Authority is often minimal. In contrast, almost nowhere in medicine is the power of Authority more absolute than for the anesthesiologist in the moments just before taking total control of the patient's vital functions. Imagine, for example, an anesthesiologist beginning to slowly administer a sedative to a patient on the table, and instead of pointlessly asking him or her to count backward, saying: "Soon I will assume control of your breathing...and as you begin to get drowsy...and eventually, go comfortably…safely asleep…you can know that your body will keep your blood inside your vessels…no bleeding…just a dry field…that's right. And when you wake…you will experience delightfully surprising comfort…surprising you, your nurses…your doctors…just comfort. And," continuing as eyelids now close and breathing slows, "during the hours and days after surgery…your body will experience really rapid wound healing… really rapid wound healing…." All that we have so far studied in the Exquisite Art assures us that the results of this intervention, in which the anesthesiologist has maximal Authority, will be hemostasis, post-operative comfort and rapid wound healing.

But if you are not the surgeon or anesthesiologist, if you are wielding neither blade nor bag, what chance have you of eliciting these same responses? True, during informed consent for surgery, you could proffer these same suggestions. "On the one hand, some **patients** may have bleeding; on the other hand, patients very much like YOU CAN HAVE VIRTUALLY BLOODLESS SURGERY…A DRY FIELD…YOU CAN KEEP YOUR OWN BLOOD…." But no matter how proficient your delivery, if the anesthesiologist or surgeon later says, "We're going to try to keep **your bleeding** to a minimum" (which is a masked suggestion for bleeding)—all bets are off. Their Authority will likely trump yours.

So how do we achieve results like those of our imagined anesthesiologist? The answer is simple: Find a technique by which to heighten our Authority, so that our suggestions achieve pre-eminence. That technique, as it happens, is the induction and utilization of hypnotic trance.

"Hypnosis"

Unfortunately, misunderstandings about what hypnosis is, how it works and what it can do abound. Even the great masters often failed to grasp the essence of their techniques. Therefore, like so many other aspects of the Exquisite Art, we begin by clarifying our concepts.

For centuries, the way to achieve "suggestive pre-eminence" has been called Hypnosis—a tragic misnomer that was wrong from its inception and has only gotten worse with time. I cringe at the use of the word, even as I delight in the use of the method. The term "hypnotisme" was probably first used in the 1820s in France, shortly after the death of Anton Mesmer. It derives from the Greek "hypnos," meaning sleep—which is not what happens in hypnotic trance. Over time, "hypnosis" became conflated with both the method of trance induction and trance itself.

To make matters worse, the occurrence of so-called hypnotic phenomena (e.g., catalepsy, anesthesias, etc.) was mistakenly thought to depend entirely on the presence of an ill-defined "trance" state. Thus, imprecise phrases like "I put him in hypnosis," or "I hypnotized him" came to be bandied about by experts, as if there was some clear and generally accepted definition of these terms. There was not. In fact, entire textbooks on hypnosis and trance have been written without ever really defining the terms in their titles.

When definitions were offered, they were invariably flimsy and ill-fitting. For example, hypnosis or hypnotic trance was often defined as "a heightened state of suggestibility in which the subject's critical faculties are suspended." But what does that really mean? And how do you recognize it? "Heightened," above what? "State of suggestibility"—define "state," define "suggestibility." "Critical faculties suspended"—if so, then why isn't every suggestion accepted by every "hypnotized" subject, instead of some suggestions being accepted by some subjects and other suggestions being accepted by other subjects? Moreover, how does hypnotic trance differ from the various religious trances into which people all over the world lapse, whether Hindu, Christian, Taoist, etc.? Or, from the curious states into which psychotics sometimes fall?

And what of the extraordinary responses (like those described in this book) by some subjects to waking suggestion? Since there were no clear definitions, pundits in the "hypnosis" camp coined terms like "non-trance hypnosis" to account for such behaviors, whereas those from the "trance" camp insisted that waking subjects who responded to suggestions were in a "trance-like state." Thus, the terms "hypnosis, trance, non-trance hypnosis and trance-like state" all emerged as ill-defined labels for otherwise unexplained phenomena—one messy terminological mumbo-jumbo, spread throughout a vast literature, spanning centuries.

Sadly, this twisted taxonomy explains nothing, offers no prospect for expansion and experimentation and is ultimately stultifying. Worse, misconceiving hypnosis actually provides spurious cover for Authorities to misspeak. "Why should it matter what we say?" they might protest: "It's not as if the patient is hypnotized or something."

For example, instead of saying to a patient with a viral syndrome, "Call me tomorrow, and let me know how well you're doing," a misguided caregiver might feel entirely justified in saying: "It will probably take you four to seven days to get well, so just hunker down and tough it out." Similarly, instead of saying to a presurgical patient, "I have many patients like **you** who wake from a successful surgery feeling comfortable and who heal very rapidly," an unaware but compassionate surgeon might say: "You'll probably have some pain and recover somewhat slowly, most do, but we'll get you through it." Not knowing that they are actually doing hypnosis (How could they know that?), caregivers of all stripes squander countless opportunities to exert positive influences on their patients.

But we're getting ahead of ourselves. Remember, we are in search of a method to magnify our persuasive power, especially when we begin with little, if any, influence. History teaches us that the object of our quest is somehow intertwined in trance and hypnosis. But how? To find out, we need a few simple answers to a few simple questions: What is trance and what is hypnosis? Are they the same? Or are they different? And if different, how so?

Let's begin our quest with an examination of trance—what is it and what role does it play in causing suggestions to actualize? Once hypnotic trance is understood and defined, we will proceed to examine the Hypnotic Method and thereby discover what hypnosis really is and what it is not.

Trance

I recently had lunch with a renowned hypnotherapist and described to him my observation that patients in the ED *in extremis* respond exactly like patients in hypnotic trance. "But don't you find," he asked, "that those patients are actually in a sort of trance themselves?" The old familiar muddle. "How do you define trance?" I asked, explaining that I didn't want to get into a conversation where the word "trance" represented one thing to me and another to him. "Well, surely there is a unique state," he said, "characterized by facial flaccidity, pallor and upward eye-rolling that only happens under hypnosis." Not really, I thought; in fact, the very opposite can also be hypnotically induced with equal ease. All I need to do is suggest to an entranced subject that they have just stepped in dog excrement, and their eyes will roll down, their face contort and their cheeks blush. Moreover, in my own experience dealing with hundreds of patients *in extremis*, I have observed no such telltale indicators of trance. Finally, any objective perusal of the literature on hypnosis reveals that trance is defined differently by virtually every author who has ever written on the subject, and very few of those definitions agree with my dear friend's definition:

1. Mesmer's "animal magnetism" trances have been described as follows:

"The reactions of patients to these means of magnetizing and treatment were not as stereotyped as the procedures; in fact, they were extremely variable. Some were calm.... Others expectorated, coughed and felt some slight pain; they might perspire and experience a local or general warmth. There were some who produced violent convulsions.... The profound repose shown by a portion of the patients was as surprising as the convulsions in another group.... All are under the influence of the magnetizer, who has a great power which he uses to dominate and agitate them."

2. Here is the description of trance provided by James Esdaile, M.D. who in 1846 published his dramatic report of 73 major and minor surgeries performed painlessly, without chemical anesthesia.

"*Flexibility of the limbs till moved, and their remaining rigid in any position we put them in, are characteristic of trance: but there are exceptions.... It sometimes happens, that the limbs become rigid as they lie, and on bending them they have always a disposition to return to a state of spasmodic extension. At other times, there is a complete relaxation of the whole muscular system.... The eyes are usually closed, but the eyelids are sometimes seen a little separated, or half-open and tremulous, and the eye is even occasionally wide open, fixed, and insensible to the light.... I have seen no symptom of congestion of the blood on the brain; the circulation in the trance being usually quite natural, like that of a sleeping person.*"

3. In 1884, the great Hippolyte Bernheim, M.D., published one of the finest volumes in the field, entitled *Hypnosis and Suggestion*. Here is his description of trance:

"*Some subjects experience only a more or less pronounced dullness, a heaviness in the lids, and sleepiness.... In some cases, somnolence...cannot be induced, but the eyelids remain closed and the patients cannot open them.... The lids are as if cataleptic.... I repeated, 'Try to open them.' She used all her force of will without succeeding, until I brought the charm to an end by saying, 'You may open them.' In the second degree.... The limbs passively retain the positions in which they are placed.... If this is not sleep, it is at least a peculiar psychical condition which diminishes the force of cerebral resistance, and which renders the mind receptive to suggestion. In the third degree...the patient is capable of making automatic movements. I move both arms, one about the other. I say, 'You cannot stop.' The arms keep up the rotation.... The fourth degree is characterized...by the loss of relationship with the outer world.... His senses are only in communication with the operator.... The fifth and sixth degrees...forgetfulness, upon waking, of all that has happened during sleep—constitute somnambulism.... The patient remains asleep according to the operator's will, becoming a perfect automaton, obedient to all his commands.... I add that docility to suggestion and the ease with which diverse phenomena are provoked, are not always in proportion to the depth of hypnotic sleep.... Each sleeper has, so to speak, his own individuality, his own special personality. I only wish to emphasize that the aptitude for realizing suggestive phenomena is not always proportional to depth of the sleep."*

4. Here is Freud, writing in 1891:

"First the patient's face assumes a rigid look, his breathing deepens, his eyes grow moist and blink frequently, one or more swallowing movements occur, and finally the eyeballs turn inwards and upwards, the eyelids fall and hypnosis is there."

5. Bandler and Grinder, who were students of Milton Erickson, M.D., in 1981 wrote:

"In trance there is a flattening or a flaccidity of the muscles in the face, and there is a symmetry which is uncharacteristic of the waking state.... Any unconscious movements—jerky, involuntary kinds of shudder movements—are really good indicators of a developing trance state...and when they go into an altered state, whatever breathing pattern is characteristic for them will change.... Especially as you get into the deeper stages of trance, there will be muscle relaxation and an increased flow of blood in the extremities.... If the eyes roll all the way up in the head, that's a good indicator of a fairly deep trance. However, lots of people go into a profound trance with their eyes open..., and in addition, there will be many other changes that you can observe which will be unique to the person you are working with."

As I said, trance is described differently by different authors. Nevertheless, there are some common elements in this historical medley. First, and this is more evident when you read the entirety of the texts, the terms "trance" and "hypnosis" are almost invariably mixed and muddled. Second, however ill-defined, all authors in one way or another acknowledge the "great power" or influence of trance. And third, the operator's tacit and express suggestions definitely elicit responses, often non-ordinary and non-voluntary, which are reflected in the subject's face, eyes, breathing and musculature.

But isn't every mental and physical state, every recollection or fantasy, associated with a certain configuration of the face, eyes, breathing and musculature? So, again, what is so unique about hypnotic trance?

Allow me this brief metaphor:

You meet a friend and colleague, someone every bit your equal, for lunch in the city. He is an outdoorsman; you are pure city folk. He invites you to go backpacking in the mountains. "Don't worry," he says. "I've been up there a hundred times. We'll hike, fish, stargaze. It'll be great."

And so, all geared-up and ready, you begin the adventure. Soon you are deep in the woods. It is beautiful, albeit unfamiliar. But your friend knows exactly where you are and where you are going. Together, you press onward—deeper, farther. You can no longer tell north from south, but he knows the way. You follow. A storm looms. Under the lowering sky, you pitch your tents and huddle up. Your friend remains calm and confident, no big deal. The storm rages through the night.

The next morning, under clear skies, you are off again; but in the slick mud, you turn your ankle. In seconds, it swells like a plum. You try standing, but the pain is piercing. "What now?" you plead. The forest surrounds you, a fog is descending. You are helpless and dependent.

Now, let me ask: Your friend and colleague, is he still every bit your equal? Or, is he now endowed by circumstance with Authority? Will you challenge his answer, in the depths of the forest, as you might have challenged his answer back home?

And what if he happens to answer your "What now?" with: "I'll wrap your ankle with this elastic bandage and lay on my hands the way an old Yaqui healer once taught me. Then, despite your doubts or fears, that ankle will become surprisingly comfortable, and we will both stand up and walk out of here. I guarantee it."

Isn't it now clear that his suggestions—in the depths of your dependency— might very well come to pass, at least in part?

It is a fitting metaphor. For this much we know: During a "hypnotic" encounter, the "operator" guides and the "subject" agrees (tacitly or expressly) to follow. The experience is unusual and often disorienting, especially at first. It is like the unfamiliar forest. Led by a skilled operator, conscious self-instigated behaviors become fewer and fewer: your own volition becomes, as it were, supplanted by the will of the operator/guide. Soon, there is **a paucity of non-prescribed behaviors**: meaning, a relative absence of observable behaviors other than those prescribed by the operator. Whatever the hypnotist's preconception of trance, he guides you there—deeper, farther—with suggestions both expressed and implied. It is as if he now controls consciousness itself. What you see, feel, smell. But not just consciousness. The body that once only you controlled, now responds to his suggestions. The hand rises and suspends without your volitional input. The breathing slows. It is an odd world—a place of strange occurrences. And while there may have been many paths into this place called "trance," you know of only one way out: To follow him, the one who led you, The One least uncertain—the Authority.

Thus, we discover the principal purpose of trance in the clinical setting: **Trance enhances Authority.**

And how do we recognize trance? As mentioned above, externally, **the prime characteristic of hypnotic trance is a paucity of non-prescribed behaviors.** Internally, as Erickson often reminded his students, the experience of trance is unknowable (to outsiders) and idiosyncratic—dependent upon the unique personality, outlook and experience of the subject. True, there are physiologic concomitants to the internal images and memories prescribed during trance. "A peaceful field of flowers with grasses gently blowing" is likely, in many subjects, to evoke facial flaccidity, pallor and deep diaphragmatic breathing. However, the very same imagery, inadvertently offered to a hay fever sufferer, will likely produce facial contortions, flushing and rapid chest breathing. In other words, it is not the physiologic responses to suggested experiences that are determinative of trance. Rather, again, it is the **paucity of non-prescribed behaviors.**

Consider the following two cases. Each required essentially the same therapeutic suggestion. Each resulted in the same dramatic, life-saving response.

In the first case, wherein my Authority was maximal, trance was not necessary. In the second case, wherein my Authority was initially quite thin, trance was crucial.

Case 1

She is 80 years old, the mother of a movie star, in ventricular tachycardia (a cardiac arrhythmia) for the second time in her life. She knows it can kill her, especially if her blood pressure begins to fall, which it is doing. Fear is written on her face.

I see we have a little time before it becomes necessary to use electricity for cardioversion. She is frail, and I would rather spare her the trauma, if possible. I ask for lidocaine, and the nurse leaves to retrieve it. The patient and I are alone. Her blood pressure is 80/40.

"You must be somewhat nervous," I say, synchronizing my breathing with hers. "And yet, you have come out of this before. Your heart knows how to NORMALIZE ITSELF…how to be..in..a..reg..u..lar..rhy..thm,… and it can. I need you to LET THE HEART…BE JUST NORMAL…NOW."

Nothing fancy. And, honestly, no expectation or belief on my part, as this is my first attempt at treating an arrhythmia with waking suggestion.

Seconds later, the nurse returns with the medication. "Look!" she exclaims. The monitor now shows normal sinus rhythm, blood pressure 105/84.

It was different with Jimmy, a 20-year-old with congenital heart disease, who presented one night in unstable atrial flutter with progressively declining blood pressure. Jimmy had known doctors all his life, and they had been wrong more often than right. When he was born, his parents were told Jimmy probably would not make it out of the nursery. From that day on, doctors lacked absolute Authority.

Case 2

It is the end of a long shift in the ED. Dr. Edwin Yager, from UCSD, has been shadowing me, observing the Exquisite Art in practice. One of my Emergency Physician colleagues asks, "Steve, I've tried multiple medications on Jimmy," we all knew Jimmy from his many ED visits, "all to no avail. Before we have to electrically cardiovert him, you think you could give hypnosis a shot?" I want to decline. I am spent. But the indomitable Dr. Yager (25 years my elder) prevails, "Let's do it, Steve. It could be fun."

Like most artists, Jimmy (a musician) is easy to induce. While in trance, I offer suggestion after suggestion: direct, indirect, metaphors, complex dissociations—a full bag of tricks. Nothing is working. Dr. Yager looks on expectantly. The monitor shows atrial flutter, unchanged. Gradually, Jimmy's blood pressure is declining.

"...and I want you to know, Jimmy," I offer, all but giving up "...that you can take all the time you need in the next 3 to 4 minutes... to wake up...knowing you can only do so...once you have comfortably **find the way __ return to normal,** *regular rhythm...only waking with everything normal." (sic) My final strategy, a double bind. (NOTE: the syntax violation, found > find, allows me to embed the suggestion.)*

Minutes pass...Jimmy's eyelids flutter, subtle movements return to his face, and then just before waking—there it is: normal sinus rhythm! Dr. Yager is delighted. I am relieved and exhausted. "So how do you feel?" I ask. "I think I did it," a wide-awake Jimmy says triumphantly.

"...and you can, JIMMY, DO IT AGAIN WHENEVER YOU NEED TO," I add.

There are three important lessons here.

The first is **trance is not necessary when Authority is maximal.** In such cases, you can evoke non-ordinary, non-voluntary responses with simple commands.

A patient *in extremis,* an accident victim on the side of the road, an injured senior in your charge—anyone who finds themselves helpless and dependent is scanning for The One least uncertain. If you are that One, "Your Reality = Their Reality."

Second, when Authority is limited, **trance enhances Authority.** That is exactly why I chose to induce a trance in Jimmy's case. While I didn't need the additional Authority with the movie star's mother, I most certainly did need it with the ever-skeptical Jimmy. Again, trance—whose external hallmark is a paucity of non-prescribed behaviors—enhances Authority.

Third, **the influence of the Authority does not end when the trance ends.** In Jimmy's case, the most important suggestion came not during but *after* the trance. As he later attested, this post-trance suggestion ("…and you can, JIMMY, DO IT AGAIN WHENEVER YOU NEED TO") gave Jimmy control over his dysrhythmia for the remainder of his life. If hypnosis were trance and trance were hypnosis, there would be no reason to append this final suggestion. The moment of influence would have passed. Imagine if, after Jimmy awoke, saying, "I think I did it," I had replied: "Or the hypnosis did. But don't worry, we can always use hypnosis next time, too." That careless retort, predicated on the mistaken notion that when trance ends, so does the operator's influence, is a curse—and a potentially lethal one at that.

* * *

Let's summarize our discussion so far. We acknowledge there are times, due to the inherent risks of the situation (e.g., impending surgery) or our diminished Authority (e.g., the subject is a friend, family member, resistant patient), when we need tools to enhance the likelihood our suggestions will actualize. Trance is one such tool. The unfamiliarity of the experience—the non-ordinary and non-voluntary nature of the responses—creates a sense of helplessness and dependency in the subject that enhances the Authority of the operator. This is why patients in trance respond to suggestions like patients in *extremis*—both feel helpless and dependent; both subjugate their will to the will of the Authority.

To be clear:

1. **Hypnotic trance,** as I am discussing it here, involves one or more subjects and an operator. (We will leave the topic of "self-hypnosis" for another time.)

2. **The operational hallmark of hypnotic trance is the subject's paucity of non-prescribed behaviors.** Physiological manifestations are too varied and contingent to be pathognomonic of trance. This is not to say or imply that subjects are inactive within the trance. Interpretations and responses always reflect the personality, constitution and experience of the subject. Suggesting hand levitation, for example, often leaves it to the subject to "decide" which hand, how high, at what speed and for how long the hand shall stay suspended. In this important sense, Erickson was right to emphasize that subjects always react "idiosyncratically." But the dominant, externally observable feature of hypnotic trance is that the subject's idiosyncratic responses operate, for the most part, within the confines of behaviors prescribed by the operator.

3. **The principal use of trance in the clinical setting is to enhance Authority,** to increase the likelihood that the operator's suggestions will actualize.

As your Authority is enhanced through trance, you become more and more capable of deepening the trance—meaning, more and more capable of eliciting increasingly non-normal, non-voluntary responses. The great hypnotists thus advanced by increments: asking first for slightly non-normal responses, waiting for those responses to manifest thereby enhancing their Authority, and then using that enhanced Authority to ask for yet more non-normal, non-voluntary responses, and so on.

It is critical for Artful Caregivers to understand that once the trance is over, Authority does not automatically revert to its pre-trance status; in fact, as we saw with the case of Jimmy, the residual Authority of the operator post-trance offers a fertile opportunity for planting additional salutary suggestions.

4. **Trance is not hypnosis** (which I will define shortly). Rather, **trance is a complex, aggregate response** to suggestions. I often demonstrate this to

medical students by inducing a trance and then suggesting that the subject experience hand levitation and catalepsy, glove anesthesia, and hemostasis. I confirm this by placing a needle through a vein on the dorsum of the elevated hand, without the subject evincing pain or bleeding. Then, I awaken the patient with the suggestion, "…allowing yourself to become fully awake and alert, even as the hand remains afloat…a hand, you can forget to feel…even as you continue to keep your blood." The subject then awakens and engages with others in an easy colloquial manner. Meanwhile, the hand remains numb and afloat, the needle bloodlessly piercing the vein. Trance does not cause catalepsy, anesthesia or hemostasis. Rather, trance is one effect of many, each in response to suggestion.

The force that drives those suggestions to actualization is still in effect, even after the trance has ceased. We know Authority is a component of that force. The question is: Is it Authority alone, or are there other component forces we have yet to discover that compel subjects to comply?

***

It turns out there are other component forces that can drive our suggestions to actualization. The prodigious Authority of the early hypnotists eclipsed these lesser forces, and so, contributed greatly to the initial confusion regarding hypnosis. Only in modern times, with the work of Milton Erickson and his astute observers John Grinder and Richard Bandler, have these ancillary components emerged from the shadows as important elements of the Hypnotic Method. Let's now turn to an examination of those ancillary components. As you will see, our efforts here are about to yield some surprising answers to the question: What is Hypnosis?

The Hypnotic Method

If trance is sometimes necessary to enhance our Authority, how do we induce trance when we do not have adequate Authority to command it? And again, as we asked at the beginning of this chapter, how can we induce other complex responses (e.g., rapid wound healing, sustained pain relief, tumor regression) when our Authority is minimal?

These are the questions Milton Erickson posed, in some form or fashion, early in his career. His time and place in history did not endow him with the august stature of the early hypnotists, so he could not simply command his wary psychiatric patients into trance. Instead, the former polio victim who was once confined to an iron lung pursued his fascination with the subtleties of verbal and nonverbal communication, eventually developing ingenious methods for circumventing resistance and driving suggestions to actualization.

Let's look at a classic example of an Authoritarian power-induction, and then contrast it with Erickson's ingenious Hypnotic Method.

First, here is the great Hippolyte Bernheim, M.D., describing his method of trance induction in 1884:

"If necessary, I hypnotized one or two patients in his presence.... When I have thus banished from his mind the...fear that attaches to that unknown condition, above all when he has seen patients cured or benefited (sic)...then I say, 'Look at me and think of nothing but sleep. Your eyelids begin to feel heavy, your eyes tired. They begin to wink, they are getting moist, you cannot see distinctly. They are closed.'"

Now, contrast this with the artful insinuations and subtle behaviors of Erickson, circa 1952:

"...When she had settled herself to her satisfaction, she remarked that she would like to smoke a cigarette. She was immediately given one, and she proceeded to smoke lazily, meditatively watching the smoke drifting upward. Casual conversational remarks were offered about the pleasure of smoking, of watching the curling smoke, the feeling of ease in lifting the cigarette to her mouth, the inner sense of satisfaction of becoming entirely absorbed just in smoking comfortably and without need to attend to any external things. Shortly, casual remarks were made about inhaling

and exhaling, these words timed to fit in with her actual breathing. Others were made about the ease with which she could almost automatically lift her cigarette to her mouth and then lower her hand to the arm of the chair. These remarks were also timed to coincide with her actual behavior. Soon, the words "inhale," "exhale," "lift," and "lower" acquired a conditioning value of which she was unaware because of the seemingly conversational character of the suggestions. Similarly, casual suggestions were offered in which the words sleep, sleepy, and sleeping were timed to her eyelid behavior."

Bernheim's suggestions are driven almost entirely by his Authority: his reality becomes the subject's reality; his will becomes the subject's will. In his day, he was nothing more—and nothing less—than the modern version of the Asclepian priest. His results nothing more—and, again, nothing less—than the Placebo Effects of a complex and credible ritual. Or, if you like, the actualized commands of a physician whose desperately dependent patients had no choice but to view him as the absolute Authority.

We should note that Bernheim's technique still works…just not on everyone. As mentioned earlier, I have entranced dozens of children with the following sentence: "I want you to TRY…just TRY [I say this while flashing first one finger, then two, then one…] to stay awake for just one…I mean two [fingers still flashing back and forth]…more minutes." True, I use confusion to focus their attention, and the clever connotation of the word "try" to indirectly suggest sleep. But beneath it all, this is a power-induction. It works owing to the child's awareness of my Authority as conferred by the parents. That same induction is unlikely to work on a friend or suspicious colleague.

On the other hand, Authority contributes only faintly to Erickson's method (at least, initially). Instead, Erickson relies on two other compelling patterns, which once established, tend to drive suggestions to actualization. These two patterns, *Rapport* and Linkage, are at the core of the modern Hypnotic Method and constitute vital elements in the Exquisite Art of Caregiving.

Let's begin with the fundamental principle behind the **Hypnotic Method.** It is a principle at once both sublimely simple and profoundly powerful.

Patterns Persist

This is the simple principle upon which all human communication rests, including the Hypnotic Method. Today, the principle finds expression in the exciting field of neuroplasticity, as: "neurons that fire together, wire together." But this is nothing new. Lucretius (first century, B.C.) wrote: "When patterns are established more or less, even from the beginning of the world, they tend to keep that order and recurrence." And writing in 1890, William James affirmed: "When two elementary brain-processes have been active together or in immediate succession, one of them, on reoccurring, tends to propagate its excitement into the other." Some 36 years after James, the eminent Russian physiologist I.P Pavlov enunciated the same principle, commenting on "…impulses which on repetition tend to follow the same path, and so establish conditioned reflexes." Whatever the anatomic substrate, again, Patterns Persist.

For example:

- Verbal Patterns Persist: Think of the stutterer, who breaks a verbal pattern with his stuttering. Your urge is to complete it. "I h-had a g-great g-golf day…h-hit a h-hole in wa-wa-wa—" "One!" you blurt, completing the "hole in one" pattern you are familiar with. Or, recall my simple method for painless injections: "Try to not say what I don't say: Oh say can you _____, by the dawn's early _____," using first confusion (e.g., a double negative), and then the first words of the United States' national anthem, but omitting "see" and "light."
- Visual Patterns P rsist: You just completed one, and now here is anoth r. (sic) I am assuming here that you completed the words "persist" and "another."
- Auditory Patterns Persist: A song is cut off on the radio, mid-verse. You complete it "in your head."

- Behavioral Patterns Persist: This is called "conditioning" or "association."

Three dominant patterns comprise the Hypnotic Method, each varying in strength from case to case and moment to moment. They are Authority, *Rapport* and Linkage.

Authority

We have already devoted considerable time and effort to exploring the power and reach of this important ("My Reality = Your Reality") pattern. Suffice to say, it is undoubtedly hardwired in the species, triggered by helplessness and dependency, and capable of instigating profound changes—both physical and psychological. Authority, almost by definition, assures "suggestive pre-eminence" to the extent that, when it is maximal, no other patterns are necessary to drive ideas to actualization.

Rapport

A cardinal pattern in human behavior is imitation. "I = You." After all, our genetic structure is 97-98% identical to that of chimpanzees. Monkey see, monkey do. Unconsciously, we routinely imitate the behavior of others: posture, breathing, laughing, coughing, fashion, religion, politics, etc. Of course, we do not imitate everyone. But we certainly imitate more people than we know. Look, for example, at any group of people and you will see postural alignments and behavioral mimicries unwittingly taking place. It is always there. His hand rises to his chin, hers rises too. Her legs are crossed, so too are the lady's next to her. She scratches her scalp, moments later he scratches his. And so on.

Realize, this is an empirical assertion. If you doubt it, look around. Really look. Here is one classic example: You are in a theatre, deeply engrossed in the movie's tender story. A man in the front row coughs, another to the side follows, soon two or three more people are coughing. Why? Because they are in *Rapport*—seeing the same images, feeling the same emotions, hearing the same music, sitting in the same attitude: the pattern is formed ("I = You"),

Rapport. And, once the pattern is formed, it tends to persist. The same is true of contagious laughter and yawning—Patterns (in this case *Rapport*) Persist.

As Mark Twain observed in 1900:

"A person of vast consequences can introduce any kind of novelty in dress and the general world will presently adopt it—moved to do it, in the first place, by the natural instinct to passively yield to that vague something recognized as authority, and in the second place by the human instinct to train with the multitude and have its approval.... We are creatures of outside influences; as a rule we do not think, we only imitate."

So much wisdom in one plain paragraph: "...the natural instinct to passively yield to...authority" and "...to train with the multitude..." Stunning.

Equally stunning were John Grinder and Richard Bandler who, by keenly studying Dr. Erickson in action, were able to dissect and methodize much of his technique. They called the imitative pattern, which Erickson set up with his patients, *Rapport* and the technique by which he established this pattern "Pacing" or "Mirroring." (NOTE: Here we are using *Rapport* as a technical term, denoting a calculable sameness between two or more entities, in contradistinction to the warm and fuzzy meaning of the term in the vernacular.) Hints of this fundamental pattern, *Rapport*, range back in the hypnosis literature from Meares to Mesmer and beyond. But, nowhere is it better explicated than in the work of Grinder and Bandler:

"But if you gauge the tempo of your voice to the rate of their breathing, if you blink at the same rate that they blink, if you nod at the rate that they're nodding, if you rock at the same rate that they're rocking...you will build rapport."

Once the *Rapport* pattern ("I = You") is established, it has momentum: meaning, a tendency to self-perpetuate...to persist. For example, if I were to lift my hand and scratch my neck, anyone in *Rapport* with me would soon (after a brief lag period, 15–20 seconds) feel compelled to lift their hand and scratch their neck, too. Grinder and Bandler referred to this phenomenon as Pacing (i.e., the imitative phase) and Leading (i.e., when a non-imitative behavior is initiated and thereafter mimicked by those in *Rapport*).

"You can use nonverbal pacing and leading either by itself, or as a part of another induction. I recommend that at some point you practice just the nonverbal portion. Without words, just arrange yourself in a mirroring position," meaning establish *Rapport*. *"Then you can very slowly—noticing how fast the person follows you—put yourself into a deep trance."*

Here, the authors are proposing a *Rapport*-Induction: whereby you lead by going into "an altered mental state" and the subject in *Rapport* is drawn to follow. This works, but it is clearly an advanced technique that requires some level of sophistication on the part of the operator. Let's leave that for another time.

More commonly, *Rapport* is used to draw the subject into trance incrementally, using both words and deeds. For example, once *Rapport* is established, I might say:

> *"...and as you allow your eyes to remain fixed on my eyes...,"* while I fix my gaze on their eyes ("I = You")

> *"...in a moment, you might feel the eyes wanting to close...,"* as I slowly lower my eyelids ("I = You")

> *"...so that you really can begin to relax...and just let go...,"* allowing my muscles to relax and let go ("I = You"), and so forth...always building on the previous increments.

The attributes one can imitate or "pace" to establish *Rapport* are legion. Certainly, some have greater importance than others. Chief among them, in my experience, are breathing and intention. I tend to "pace" intention first, by agreeing with the subject on our shared goals. On the other hand, I often save breathing for last—after posture, movements, voice volume and cadence, blinking and head tilt...among others. Generally, I talk and listen to the subject, as I shift from mimicking one attribute to another, so as not to be obvious. (Trust is broken if your subject detects your mimicry.) If I am establishing *Rapport* as part of trance induction, I'll often delay matching a subject's breathing till after eye closure, especially if their pattern is difficult to detect and requires visual focus.

The central notion here is that if "I = You," and "I" change in some way, then "you" will change in that way, too. Why? Because Patterns Persist.

Here are four key observations about the *Rapport* pattern:

1. The Rapport Pattern Is NOT Unidirectional

This is important. Whenever the *Rapport* threshold is crossed—meaning, whenever the ability to Lead exists—the relationship becomes bidirectional. The operator/subject dyad dissolves. There is a one-ness. So, beware. As caregivers, you are likely to establish *Rapport* with people who have problems of one sort or the other. You do not want to take on those problems. As John Grinder taught me in 1985, protect yourself. How? Create within yourself a Host Defense that repudiates any and all adverse external influences. This is not difficult to do: Self-suggest such a defense, unambivalently: "Surface sameness only—nothing penetrates," is my self-suggested shield.

2. Rapport Affords the Subject a Deep Sense of Alliance

Provided the subject likes and trusts themselves, they will like and trust you to a far greater degree than they would if *Rapport* had not been established. In practical terms, when caregivers are in *Rapport* with our charges, both tend to understand that no matter what the outcome we are doing our very best. The relationship feels warm, forgiving and genuine.

3. Once Established, Rapport Needs to be Maintained

With a little practice, establishing *Rapport* takes only seconds. I do it, for example, when I first meet a patient. Maintaining the pattern throughout the session, thereafter, relies on continued subtle mimicry with special attention to the subject's breathing and intentions.

She sits on the gurney waiting. As I approach, I sense her kinetics (she sits still, breathing slowly) and I adjust my movements to hers. My head tilts as hers does. Our eyes meet and I blink as she blinks.

"Hi, I'm Dr. Bierman," I say, extending my hand. We shake hands, the force of her grip met with an equal force by me.

"I'm Janet. I'm hurting, Doctor."

"Janet, hi. You're hurting? Can you tell me where?" I say, "pacing" her words to describe her complaint. (I could have said, "Where is your pain?" But that would have distinguished us from each other—the opposite of a Rapport maneuver.)

She sighs and says, "I guess everywhere, Doctor."

I sigh, too, and ask, "Everywhere? Even down here?" I ask, pointing to her toes.

In seconds, I've paced her kinetics, sighs, verbiage, blinking. I've also begun to lead by directing my attention to her toes and asking her to follow me there. From here, it is a small step to eye closure, imagining a safe and wonderful place where you can "just rest and be comfortable...just comfortable."

4. Rapport Is an Essential Component of the Modern Hypnotic Method

Its application extends far beyond trance induction. Being in *Rapport* with someone you are caring for magnifies your persuasive influence tremendously, trance or no trance. *All that we have learned so far about the Exquisite Art— our entire toolbox—is enhanced through establishing and maintaining Rapport.* Think about it: If "I = You," then "my will = your will." My desire to have you comply with my directions, my wish for your cure, my instruction to stop bleeding, to feel comfortable, to relax—all of my intentions become your intentions, too. Thus, by establishing and maintaining *Rapport*, my ideas take on a higher likelihood of evoking their desired responses. Again, trance is one response—a complex one consisting of multiple component responses. But there are myriad other responses (e.g., relaxation, hemostasis, analgesia) Artful caregivers, by establishing and maintaining *Rapport*, can and do elicit for their patients' benefit.

Linkage

Linkage is the third compelling pattern in the Hypnotic Method. It exists when "My Words = Your Experience," which is distinctly different from *Rapport*, wherein "My Words = Your Words" (a subset of "I = You"). With Linkage, the operator is saying what the subject is experiencing, whether that experience is an idea or an action. This in mind, let's look more closely at what Erickson is doing in the induction I previously quoted:

> "...*Shortly, casual remarks were made about inhaling and exhaling, these words timed to fit in with her actual breathing. Others were made about the ease with which she could almost automatically lift her cigarette to her mouth and then lower her hand to the arm of the chair. These remarks were also timed to coincide with her actual behavior. Soon, the words "inhale," "exhale," "lift," and "lower" acquired a conditioning value of which she was unaware because of the seemingly conversational character of the suggestions.*"

What is the "conditioning" Erickson is referring to? It is Erickson's Words = His Patient's Experience. This is the Linkage pattern. Remember, Patterns Persist. If, in this moment, Erickson's words DESCRIBE what is occurring, then in the next moment, provided the pattern is established, his words can PRESCRIBE what will occur. This is why, in most trance inductions, the Linkage pattern proceeds from DESCRIBING the subject's conscious external experience to PRESCRIBING conscious internal experiences—like imagery, relaxation, etc. It is a simple formula that when coupled with *Rapport* and Authority renders an operator's suggestions virtually irresistible.

Consider this Linkage pattern, which I commonly use as part of my trance inductions:

"I would like to ask you to really focus on my eyes, so that you are seeing my eyes...and probably one a little more than the other...while I am seeing yours..."

Notice the indirection (I would like to ask you to...), then the DESCRIPTION of what the subject is likely conscious of (seeing my eyes) and probably "one a little more...," because I know there is a focal point. Of course, I am also maintaining *Rapport* by focusing on the subject's eyes. (I = You)

"And allow yourself to notice that in the center of your visual field...as you stay focused...things are always very sharp and colorful...You might notice, for example, the way the light glances off the cornea...or the colors in the iris..."

Now my words are DESCRIBING something they might not be conscious of in the moment but can quickly verify—things sharp and colorful in the center, light glancing off the cornea, colors in the iris.

"While at the far periphery...even as you stay <u>focus</u> (sic.) on the center...you can discover that things are much less distinct...much less colorful..."

I changed syntax from the expected "focused" to "focus" in order to embed the command. Then, once again, DESCRIBE a phenomenon I know they can verify. I am establishing the pattern: My words = Their experience.

"And that's a function of the retina...and it is how the great Dutch painters painted, which is why those Rembrandts seem so real..."

A very indirect suggestion to begin engaging in internal visual imagery—a subtle invitation....

"And what I would like to point out...is that a bit later...when you allow your eyes to close themselves...when they are even heavier than now...you can have the pleasure of discovering that our internal

imagery can have this same feature...central focus...peripheral indistinctness..."

Now, I am PRESCRIBING (i.e., suggesting) eyelid heaviness by saying they will get "even" heavier than they are now, and eye closure "a bit later," while also presupposing ("discovering") becoming conscious of internal imagery.

> *"And you might even allow yourself to see some pleasant image from memory or imagination or a combination...something you can, Julie, just watch and enjoy."*

More indirection ("might even allow...") to suggest internal imagery. And ending with the embedded command: "...Julie, just watch and enjoy."

At this point, provided I have also established and maintained *Rapport*, most subjects are becoming internally absorbed, and there is a noticeable paucity of non-prescribed behaviors. In other words, the subject is becoming entranced.

While it is important here to grasp what I'm saying to the subject—i.e., linking my words to their experience, as I move from describing experience to prescribing it—it is even more important to appreciate what I am NOT saying. I am not speaking in a manner that can be controverted or contested, not making falsifiable assertions. Rather, I am speaking incontrovertibly—using the permissive language we learned earlier—to create a strong LINKAGE pattern that will power my suggestions to actualization.

In this regard, a few simple reminders:

1. **Avoid mandates** (pardon the irony): Instead of "you will...," use "you might, can, could...."
2. **Don't say "don't"**: "Don't spill the milk," becomes "Can you hold onto the glass?" or "Good job keeping it level."
3. **Avoid being too specific:** "the sounds of the beach" is better than "the screeching of the gulls or crashing of the waves," as there may be no birds or waves in the subject's imagery.

4. **Name it and claim it:** Remember, your words = your subject's experience. If the door slams during a session and the subject reacts, you must name it and claim it lest the Linkage pattern be broken. "And the closing of one door, however loud or soft, can be a prelude to new doors of experience opening… comfortable experiences that you can…just enjoy."

Of course, there are many more niceties to the language of the Hypnotic Method; these are brilliantly laid out in the numerous volumes written by Bandler and Grinder, which I highly recommend. But becoming adept at the nuanced language of Ericksonian hypnosis is less important than a broad understanding of the Linkage pattern, and an earnest commitment to establishing and maintaining it by using permissive language.

As with *Rapport*, Linkage imparts momentum to your suggestions, regardless of whether you are suggesting trance or some other response. Thus, **all that we have learned so far about the Exquisite Art—our entire toolbox—is enhanced through establishing and maintaining Linkage.**

* * *

Now, imagine a patient distrusting of all caregivers, who comes to you reluctantly after an injury. You want to offer suggestions for comfort and healing. But with scant Authority, your words may or may not be effective. What do you do? Trance induction is probably not appropriate for this patient, at least not initially. Do you, therefore, let the moment pass and simply wish your new patient "good luck"? Or do you use the other components of the Hypnotic Method, *Rapport* and Linkage, to help propel your Artfully expressed ideas to actualization?

Indeed, that is exactly what you do. For example, while establishing and maintaining *Rapport*:

> *You: Well, we both know that's a pretty severe ankle sprain—*
>
> *Patient: Yeah, Doc.*

*You: And yeah, on the one hand, **some people** (right hand extending away) might take a few weeks to heal, while on the other hand (left hand indicating the patient) many people, perhaps like **you**, do surprisingly well and heal very fast.*

Patient: Um...okay.

You: And while I bet that hurt considerably when it happened—

Patient: Did it ever...

You: You might be surprised to discover how really rapidly your healing system can deliver increasing comfort and stability.... Of course, it may still hurt a bit when you stand on it—

Patient: It does—

You: And yet, it can become even more comfortable with each passing day.... (And so on, with advice on proper care of the injury.)

Hypnosis Defined

Up to this point, our discussions have delivered an operational definition of Trance and an appreciation for the three principal patterns of the Hypnotic Method. Now, let's return to our original question—What is Hypnosis?

As we have seen, all healers can produce dramatic changes with their words and gestures, when they are perceived as Authorities. Among those dramatic changes is the induction of trance. But even without trance, healers can command phenomenal physical and mental responses across a broad spectrum of conditions. The "My Reality = Your Reality" Authority pattern, which arises instinctively out of a patient's sense of helplessness and dependency, confers prodigious power over body and mind.

We now understand there are two additional patterns—*Rapport* and Linkage—which can also be enlisted to empower our suggestions. These patterns have always been there to a degree (re-read Bernheim's induction with Linkage in mind); but it was Erickson who mastered them and Bandler and Grinder who methodized their use. Even in the absence of Authority, *Rapport* and Linkage are sufficiently powerful to induce dramatic responses. Virtually all of the cases I have so far presented in this book, wherein trance was not used, involved the subtle incorporation of *Rapport* and Linkage. Additionally, when Authority is scant, *Rapport* and Linkage generate the driving force behind trance induction—which, in turn, magnifies the operator's Authority, which then joins forces with *Rapport* and Linkage to further propel ideas to actualization.

So, what is Hypnosis?

Hypnosis is simply ideas evoking responses. And, the Hypnotic Method is a refinement of everyday communication designed to increase the likelihood that expressed ideas will evoke their intended responses. As such, Hypnosis may or may not involve trance. Trance is merely an effect. Just as hemostasis, anesthesia, reversion to normal sinus rhythm—just as all the various outcomes I have reported are effects. And they are all caused by the mundane and marvelous fact that ideas, especially when presented using *Rapport*, Linkage and Authority, evoke responses.

Thus, there is Hypnosis done well, and there is Hypnosis done poorly. For caregivers, as we can now discern, Hypnosis done well is what the Exquisite Art is all about.

The Communication Continuum

We now see before us the full range of the **communication continuum**, extending from the unattended rants of schizophrenics to the rhythmic engagements of Ericksonian trance-masters, from the utter absence of refinements to the near-perfect utilization of the Hypnotic Method's propulsive force. In this light, we begin to descry the miracle that is everyday communication: Here, an idea is conceived, coded and transmitted; there, the transmission is received, decoded and responded to. Not always, of course. In fact, this sequence is almost never completed in the case of a schizophrenic's vacant rant. But it comes as close as possible to "always completed" when the transmitter is in *Rapport* with the receiver, when his or her words are tightly LINKED to the subject's experience and when the gradient between the two interlocutors awakens in the subject a primordial pattern (Authority) that insists, "My Reality (the operator) = Your Reality (the subject)."

Each step along this continuum represents a refinement of everyday communication: clarity of thought; adeptness of expression; drawing and holding attention; avoiding resistance, harmonizing rhythms and movements and meanings; underscoring; observing and ratifying responses. Each step advances toward a kind of one-ness. But not a one-ness of equals. For even *Rapport*, when it is methodized and deliberate, has a driver—a dominant intention, so to speak. And that intention is to transmit the operator's idea to the subject—not to the topsoil of their consciousness where it can be blown away by winds of doubt and disagreement; but deeper, into the subsoil where the first thought-seeds of the subject's most immutable beliefs and alliances were once planted. When a patient is *in extremis,* we can do so with an unvarnished command. When our Authority is less certain, we accomplish our task using the Exquisite Art—which we now see is the Hypnotic Method, and which we now know is nothing more and nothing less than a refinement of everyday communication.

Let's pause and let that sink in....

Summarizing the Hypnotic Method

For centuries, the Hypnotic Method has been used to: (1) induce trance, and (2) elicit other extraordinary responses. Regrettably, these two distinct phenomena have forever been conflated—the single word, Hypnosis, subsuming both. Few grasped the simple fact that the induction of trance in a subject who is initially wide-awake is itself a noteworthy process, deserving of explanation. Fewer still, have understood that so-called trance phenomena can also be elicited without trance: that non-ordinary and non-voluntary responses happen in every placebo-controlled trial; that suggestions alone (driven by Authority, Linkage and/or *Rapport*) can stop bleeding, avert pain, normalize heart rhythms; and that diseases of all sorts can be cared for, and sometimes cured, with well-crafted and well-delivered suggestions—again, with or without trance. In essence, the history of "hypnosis" from Mesmer to the present day is a history of mistaking an isolated effect (i.e., trance) for a powerful cause—namely, suggestion, driven by the momentum of patterns that must persist.

- **Hypnotic Trance** is operationally defined as a condition in which the subject exhibits a **paucity of non-prescribed behaviors.** Physiologic manifestations, once again, are not pathognomonic for trance; rather, they are concomitants of the prescribed behaviors. Moreover, while it is understood that self-instigated behaviors occur during hypnotic trance, they generally occur within the pale of prescribed behaviors.
- **Hypnosis is ideas evoking responses.**
- **Hypnotic Method is a refinement of everyday communication that increases the likelihood an operator's ideas (i.e., suggestions) will evoke their intended responses.** As such, owing to the Authority vested in caregivers by our culture, we are all using a component of the Hypnotic Method (i.e., Authority) all the time, whenever we present ideas.

Implications

Let's consider some of the consequences of this grand unraveling, for the implications of this new taxonomy extend far beyond the parochial province of "hypnosis" and into the broader world of caregiving.

1. The fog of countless confusing terminologies is lifted.
2. The mysteries of placebo, shamanic healing and other therapeutic rituals are largely solved.

3. Broad areas of innovation and experimentation in caregiving are now accessible.

4. The priorities of all healing arts must now shift—placing the Exquisite Art of Caregiving at the forefront of every discipline: traditional, complementary or alternative.

5. Vague notions about demagoguery, brainwashing, Stockholm syndrome yield to a sharper, clearer understanding and context. They are all hypnotic phenomena.

While a full explication of all these implications lies beyond the scope of this book, let's peek briefly at the first three.

Terminology

We begin with the numerous confusing terminologies that are currently in use. Two categories concern us: (1) terminology relating to Hypnosis and the Hypnotic Method, and (2) terminology relating to other disciplines in the healing arts.

As to the Hypnotic Method:

- "Hypnotize"—As the term is currently used, it is a non-sequitur. Since the Hypnotic Method is a refinement of everyday communication, the term "hypnotize" should mean of or pertaining to use of the Hypnotic Method. Instead, it is used to mean trance induction. This is inaccurate. The proper term is "Entrance." You do not "hypnotize" a person, nor do you "put him in hypnosis"; rather, you entrance a person by using the Hypnotic Method.
- "Post-hypnotic suggestion"—This term is used to denote the fulfillment of a suggestion after "hypnosis" has ended. But "hypnosis" has not ended: the influence of Authority, *Rapport* and Linkage continues and thereby carries the suggestion to fulfillment. It is trance, and only trance, that has ended. Therefore, the proper term is "Post-trance suggestion."

- "Trance-like state"—This is a term without a behavioral substrate. Those who use it commonly refer to trance as a state of heightened suggestibility, and then identify that state by the facial flaccidity, pallor and diaphragmatic breathing. "Trance-like state" is used to explain suggestibility, in the absence of these signs. The term implies that a person is only suggestible if they are in some sort of trance. This is nonsense. The fact is, people are highly susceptible to suggestion when they are (1) helpless and dependent, (2) in *Rapport* or (3) compelled by Linkage to experience what their interlocutor's words prescribe. This is not trance-like. Rather, it is the Hypnotic Method at work. Saying "trance-like state" is like saying "sound-like quality," it feels meaningful, but it isn't.

- "Non-trance Hypnosis"—This term is the original misconception inverted. Because trance was the perceived cause of suggestions actualizing, it became necessary to explain the manifold responses occurring outside of trance. We now know that non-trance hypnosis IS Hypnosis (call it "waking Hypnosis" if you wish), and that trance is just one of the myriad responses Hypnosis can elicit.

As to Other Disciplines:

- Guided Imagery, Talk Therapy, Visualization, Affirmation, etc.— Therapies of this nature all involve refinements of everyday communication—ideas evoking responses—and so, they are all hypnotic therapies. Whether trance is involved depends, of course, on how trance is defined. But if you adhere to our definition, you will frequently observe these techniques invoking hypnotic trance—and, thus, magnifying the operator's Authority. Certainly, the more they employ the refinements and patterns of the Hypnotic Method, the more successful they will be in evoking their intended therapeutic responses.

Placebo, Shamanic Healing and other Therapeutic Rituals

In this connection, the following case histories will be instructive.

A. Burn Wounds

In my early days as an Emergency Physician using hypnosis, I discovered I could comfort burn patients and accelerate their wound healing by offering the following suggestion while they were in trance: "...and the wound can remain cool and comfortable...long after the trance is over." Clearly, this is a post-trance suggestion. My notion was that "cool" would result in a diminished post-injury inflammatory response—which, if not prevented, often worsens the original injury.

I was proud of this discovery, and after a series of 20 patients, shared my excellent results with the renowned hypno-surgeon Dr. Dabney Ewin. Dabney had considerable experience dealing with burn wound patients and had published on the subject. After listening attentively, he put his hand reassuringly on my shoulder and said, "But that's wrong. It's WARM and comfortable. The 'warm' suggestion brings blood to the wound and accelerates healing."

I felt terrible...until I refocused on my results. They were real. "Cool" was working, too.

B. Migraine Headaches

A few years later, while studying for the hypnosis boards, I came across two studies on the hypnotic treatment of migraine headaches.

In the first study, patients were entranced and trained to make the hand on the opposite side of their headaches icy cold. They were given the post-trance suggestion that whenever they felt a migraine coming on they could sit down, cool their hand and avert the headache. It was argued that "cool" would constrict the vessels involved and prevent the dilatory phase of the migraine—the phase thought, at the time, to be associated with the actual headache.

In the second study, subjects in trance were asked to experience warmth in both hands. The thought being that they were learning vasodilatation, which they could transfer to intracranial vessels during "the constrictive phase" of a developing migraine. These volunteers were given the post-trance suggestion to allow their hands to warm at the first inkling of a headache.

Once again, I had discovered conflicting therapeutic suggestions. Once again, both suggestions worked.

In all four instances, the desired response was achieved. The question is, how could these contradictory suggestions have all been therapeutically successful? What is the common thread?

Traditional Western medicine, as you might imagine, would dismiss these cases as instances of Placebo Effect, worthy of no further consideration—as inferior, one might say, as the methods of any charlatan or quack. On the other hand, we now understand that these Placebo Effects are, in fact, hypnotic responses—meaning, responses driven by refinements of everyday communication that include the patterns of Authority, Linkage and *Rapport*. In both burns and migraines, we may surmise that some blend of Authority, Linkage and *Rapport* conspired to drive the suggestions to actualization. But what suggestions? It defies logic to suppose that both warming and cooling can have the same effect. What is really going on?

To understand, we need to look beneath the specific interventions. There we find what I have previously called the Generic Placebo Suggestion, namely: If (X)—you submit to this ritual, then (Y)—you will experience the prescribed outcome. This is implicit. The explicit suggestions for either warmth or coolness are important, but primarily insofar as they lend credibility to (X), the ritual, and thereby do not diminish Authority. (It is, of course, possible that one or another of these interventions also holds intrinsic value.) Remember, in order <u>not</u> to undermine Authority, a well-constructed Therapeutic Ritual must:

- Be credible at the outset.
- Be somewhat difficult to achieve, but achievable.
- Remain credible upon completion.

In all cases above, these three criteria were satisfied. Additionally, in all cases, the Generic Placebo Suggestion was conveyed with sufficient momentum (i.e., Patterns Persist) to compel actualization.

This same implicit suggestion is operative in virtually all placebo-controlled clinical trials, Shamanic Healings, and other culturally accepted Therapeutic Rituals around the world.

Instead of regarding Placebo Effects with disdain, our new understandings teach us that such effects lie at the very heart of caregiving.

Innovation and Experimentation

Understanding what Hypnosis is and how it works raises numerous questions, many of which are amenable to scientific investigation. In Appendix II, I will elaborate a program of research that I believe could set Noetic Medicine on a firmer evidentiary footing, and thereby introduce it into the mainstream of the healing arts. Of course, as with all experimental science, the devil will be in the details. More on that later. For now, let's imagine an experiment roughly along the following lines:

> As suggested at the beginning of this chapter, maximal Authority resides in the anesthesiologist at the time of induction of anesthesia. Therefore, what better arena in which to scientifically test our central thesis of Authority driving ideas to actualization?

> Surgical patients, all undergoing the identical procedure, are randomly assigned to either the "count backward" group or the "suggestion" group. The former are asked to "count backward" while an intravenous sedative (like, midazolam) is administered just prior to surgery; the latter group, as the sedative is infused, are offered direct suggestions to (1) "keep your blood," (2) "wake with delightfully surprising comfort" and (3) "expe-

rience really rapid wound healing." The primary outcomes would be such measures as estimated or actual blood loss, post-operative analgesic medication usage and time to return to work (or some other objective measure of healing).

Think of the potential benefits for patients and payors alike, should the results of this experiment prove what logic and experience lead us to expect: namely, fewer infections and other complications, more rapid recoveries and diminished requirements for analgesic medication—all demonstrated in one simple clinical trial.

Summing Up

In closing this chapter, I think it is appropriate to ask: Why are humans so susceptible to suggestion? The straight answer is, we don't yet know. I strongly suspect that as brain science advances, neural or energetic systems and configurations will be delineated that more precisely define the patterns we have been discussing. Perhaps then we will be able to explain the true nature of human suggestibility.

In the meantime, I am left to observe that Authority—the pattern whereby the ideas of The One flow indelibly into the thoughts of the other—is essential to the survival of our species. Long before language, there had to have been a mechanism whereby the learnings of the elders could be passed quickly and faithfully to the young. In some young adults—destined themselves to become leaders—those transmissions eventually subordinate to reason and volition. But in most, even in modern times, Authority reigns supreme. As Schopenhauer said: "A man can do what he will, but he cannot will what he will." Such is the nature of the human herd.

I see Linkage as a subset or derivative of Authority. In childhood, the Authority's words defined our experience—"this is hot," "that is red," "this is a ball," "that is dangerous." Patterns Persist, especially in times reminiscent of childhood, when we find ourselves once again helpless and dependent.

Rapport is a one-ness, and as such, I cannot but think of the intrauterine experience we all share: wherein her rhythms (i.e., the mother's rhythms) are my rhythms, her breath is my breath, her nutrients are my nutrients, her will is my will as there can be no other.

It is as if Nature's grand prenatal pattern of coalescence, *Rapport*, were somehow restored after birth through the Patterns of Authority and Linkage—conjured by caregivers in their practice of the Exquisite Art.

*"In Surgery, the benefits of Mesmerism are not confined to
the extinction of pain during an operation, but are
of the greatest general and particular advantage in the
after-treatment of surgical diseases."*

—James Esdaile, M.D. (1846), *Mesmerism in India*

Chapter 11:
Bloodless Surgery and Painless Recovery

Perhaps the easiest and most gratifying work I do is presurgical hypnosis. The results often defy expectations, and the thankful outpourings from patients are memorable and heartwarming.

This simple procedure incorporates many of the advanced elements of the Hypnotic Method so, whether your practice offers this specific application or not, the study of it will prepare you for a broad range of situations that arise in the course of caregiving. For example, in addition to utilizing what we have already learned about *Rapport*, Linkage and Authority, the protocol for presurgical hypnosis teaches: building response potential, seeding ideas, post-trance suggestions and anticipatory (future) Linkage. The integration of these skills, along with learning this simple trance induction, will advance you mightily in the Exquisite Art.

Let me urge you to go easy on yourself, especially at first. This protocol is laden with learnings, polite pilferings from the masters and artful innovations. We all forget parts and pieces (myself included), accidentally misspeak, and often find in one session ample room for improvement in the next. Much of what is included in this protocol you already know from the preceding chapters—namely, how to elegantly convey ideas to avoid resistance, encode emphasis and elicit results. Now we are adding trance induction, maintenance and post-trance suggestions, and throwing in a little "flavor" on top of all that.

When practicing this method, take heart in knowing that even if you only get a small fraction of this right, your patients' surgeries will go better—perhaps, far better—than they otherwise would have gone. Have fun with it. And be prepared to be amazed.

Scheduling

When a patient calls to request presurgical hypnosis, let your first question be: When is the surgery? Then, schedule the one and only session you will need the evening before the procedure (or as close to that date as possible). Patients will often plead for more than one session or to be seen earlier. Trust me, resist. There are two reasons for this tactic. First, the patient will see very few people between seeing you and having the surgery; therefore, your influence is less likely to be corrupted. Second, the patient's sense of helplessness and dependency will be cresting in those final hours before the operation, and consequently your Authority will be maximal. This is what Erickson called "building response potential."

Before the Trance

Bear in mind, hypnosis (ideas evoking responses) is happening all the time—from your first words and gestures to your last. Therefore, the moment the patient enters, it begins.

Rapport

You greet them at the door and begin to mirror their head tilt, eye blink, voice volume, handshake pressure, words ("Hello" is met with "Hello," "Hi" is met with "Hi"); they sit, you sit—same attitude. Always shifting your focus from one attribute to another, so your mimicry goes undetected: Retaining enough "you" to be authentic, mirroring enough "them" to establish and maintain *Rapport*.

Linkage

"So here we are…," you begin, incontrovertibly. Taking the history, you listen attentively, crafting your replies to describe their experience. Remember, Your Words = Their Experience. For example, the evening before your patient's hip replacement surgery:

Patient: It hurts every night and wakes me two or three times a night, if not more.

You: So, I imagine you must be somewhat tired almost every day.

> NOTE: Hard to controvert (a) what you "imagine," (b) "somewhat" tired and (c) "almost" every day.

Patient: So tired.

You: So tired…I bet even a little truly comfortable sleep will be a welcome thing.…

> NOTE: Seeding, or introducing, the idea of comfort during "sleep"; and getting agreement to go there.

Patient: Definitely.

Agreement on Goals

Taking the history need not be extensive, but you should uncover any anxieties, previous surgical successes or mishaps, curses (from other Authorities) and concerns. Once this is accomplished, it is time to agree on goals. Remember, this is a *Rapport* maneuver, as shared intention is a potent component of the "I = You" *Rapport* pattern. I usually volunteer what I know to be the three shared goals of all surgical patients (see below) and then ask what additional goals there might be. Often, the patient adds some characteristic (e.g., beauty or agility) or faculty (e.g., sexual function or bladder control) they wish to retain.

You: So, I understand you've had a certain degree of anxiety, which is natural. And yet, we can probably both agree that if you knew your procedure would be successful—that you would not lose blood, that your wounds would heal really rapidly and that you would wake from surgery with delightfully surprising comfort—if you knew all that to be true, wouldn't you be able to...JANE, RELAX A LOT MORE?

Patient: I think so...yes.

You: I think so, too. And so, what you might take comfort in knowing... is that while you have a conscious mind—and that mind can think and reason and doubt and wonder—you also have an unconscious mind...

Patient: Uh-huh...

You: And just as your conscious mind is the result of millions of years of evolution, so too is your unconscious mind—which is what hypnosis recruits and utilizes. Millions of years of evolving...with one and only one purpose...to protect you.

> NOTE: This may or may not be true. Students of hypnosis regularly mistake suggestions for facts, especially when they are offered outside of trance. What matters here is that this suggestion sets the frame whereby the unconscious forces we are about to enlist are protective and only protective.

You: I often think of what it must have been like for ancient humans... far from the village, foraging, hunting.... Of course, there were cuts and joint dislocations and wounds of all sorts. They had to have a way TO KEEP YOUR BLOOD from being lost, to stop the hurt...to FORGET TO FEEL...and to HEAL REALLY RAPIDLY.... The survival of the species depended on it.... And so, the unconscious had to evolve mechanisms to DO THIS. (Note the UNDERSCORING.)

Patient: I suppose that makes sense.

You: I suppose, too...and so, if you agree, let's let our goals include what the unconscious is actually designed to do…and what it wants to do…

Patient: Yes, definitely.

You: And let's definitely remember that the best way to instruct the unconscious is with positive suggestions. Rather than say, "Don't spill the milk," for example, we say, "Keep the glass level."

> NOTE: This is a critical point. Patients will often state their goal, initially, in the negative: "I don't want to…." It is important to take the time and work with them to restate that goal in positive terms.

Patient: Okay.

You: So instead of saying "Don't bleed," let's agree to "keep your own blood" inside your vessels. Surgeons call this a dry field.

Patient: Dry field?

You: Yes, the field is the area in which they operate. The hip area in your case. So, dry as a bone.

Patient: Okay.

You: Now, it happens that the unconscious is so good at keeping your blood that we have to allow one small exception.

Patient: What's that?

You: That's when the lab technician comes, before or after surgery, to draw blood from a vein in your arm. Let's let the unconscious understand that it can LET THE LAB TECHNICIAN HAVE THE BLOOD THEY NEED FOR LAB TESTS.

> NOTE: Including this exception is essential. Recall, I learned this lesson the hard way after my first presurgical hypnosis patient, Jan, was stuck multiple times unsuccessfully for lab tests. You can offer this suggestion before, during and/or after trance—just be sure to offer it.

Patient: Makes sense.

You: And doesn't it also make sense to have REALLY RAPID WOUND-HEALING?

> NOTE: I always say that phrase much faster than my usual cadence, as a metaphorical suggestion of sorts.

Patient: Sure…

You: Especially since the faster it heals the safer you are.

Patient: If you say so.…

You: Well, I will also say, if your surgeon says to have the stitches out in 14 days, my experience with patients very much like you, Jane, is to schedule to have the stitches out in 11 or 12 days, but no later.

Patient: And why's that?"

You: Because with really rapid wound-healing, the wound will be healed by then. I mean you're not opposed to surprising yourself and your surgeon, are you?

Patient: No, not at all.

You: And what a nice surprise to wake from the surgery feeling comfortable. But remember, not everyone uses hypnosis to invite their unconscious to cooperate. And so, nurses and doctors are used to those other patients. On the other hand, you have a partner with enormous capacity—your unconscious. So, YOU CAN FORGET TO FEEL. *Just as, until I mention it, you probably forgot to feel the back of your left… ankle. Right?*

Patient: (Nods assent.)

You: And finally, before we begin…

> NOTE: Of course, the Artful Caregiver knows we have already begun.

"...since you are a human and I am a human, it is possible that I might accidentally misspeak. And so, it's important to know that my words are just symbols for meanings your unconscious can use to achieve our shared goals. For example, if I say 'warm' and 'cold' is better for you, then the word 'warm' can be a symbol to your unconscious for whatever temperature feels right for you..."

> NOTE: I call this a "generic disclaimer." Having now established this, from the patient's perspective, I can never misspeak.

I would ask that you give this part of the transcript a careful rereading. While it may seem like casual conversation, there is a lot of deliberate work going on. "My words = Your words" is part of the *Rapport* I am cultivating; you can see that I often begin my responses with the same words (sometimes, with minor modification) the patient has just used. Additionally, I am also covertly mirroring the patient's observable behaviors.

Also, notice that throughout, to maintain Linkage, I carefully craft statements and offer ideas using permissive language: might, can, could, etc. And, I am using eye contact and vocal modification to UNDERSCORE key suggestions. Finally, in the context of stating goals in the positive, I am also "seeding" or introducing the chief therapeutic suggestions. So, a lot is happening in this short sequence.

Again, to be effective, you certainly do not need to include every one of these elements. My hope, however, is that this transcript will guide you toward eventual mastery. Meantime, patience and practice.

Trance Induction

Not included in the above transcript is the discussion I invariably have with patients about trance, its naturalistic quality and how no conscious effort is needed: "just wait and watch and wonder."

During that discussion, I always add: "You often hear people talk about trance going deeper. But if you think about it, you are in that chair when you are just comfortable…and you are in the same chair when you are in a light trance…and you are in the exact same spatial location when you enjoy the full benefits of a deep trance…So 'deep' is just a metaphor for the unconscious becoming freer and freer…to do…to achieve. Because the conscious mind is the know-er; the unconscious is the do-er." Thus, I set the frame—this trance will be about allowing non-voluntary events to occur.

"I wonder if you could, JANE ALLOW YOUR EYES TO CLOSE THEMSELVES…not too tight…just tight enough to comfortably stay close (sic) and…allow yourself__pay attention to some things you might not have…."

> NOTE: This first sentence is worth memorizing. It (1) eludes resistance "I wonder," (2) initiates a dissociation "close themselves," (3) indirectly suggests eyelid catalepsy "not too tight…just tight enough to stay close," and (4) embeds commands—for eye closure (e.g., "close," instead of "closed") and for the patient's attention. I also use the patient's first name "Jane," to signal an embedded (UNDERSCORED) command. And, I drop the "to" in the infinitive "to pay" to embed the command: "__pay attention to some things you might not have.

Of course, once the patient has closed their eyes, it is easy to observe their breathing and to synchronize your suggestions with it. This is *Rapport* maintenance. It needn't be every breath. The breathing sets the rhythm; it is "the drumbeat of the dance."

Next, I begin to DESCRIBE certain experiences the patient is either aware of or can easily confirm. These experiences are divided into the various modalities of sensation—kinesthetic, visual, auditory. I often will add olfactory and cognitive allusions as well. As a general rule, it is useful to begin in the modality most likely to be engaged by the patient at the time. So, if the patient is staring at an object, I will begin with the visual modality; if he or she is occupied with an unpleasant feeling, I will begin with that feeling and quickly digress to other more pleasant sensations. Once a solid

LINKAGE pattern is established through these various DESCRIPTIONS, I can begin PRESCRIBING behaviors. Customarily, the initial PRESCRIBED behaviors are comfort and relaxation.

Remember, trance induction generally proceeds from description of external events to prescription of internal experiences.

Feelings

"...like certain feelings...for example, which you can think of as outside/inside feelings.... On the outside...it's nice to discover that as the eyes close, and you enjoy the soothing comfort of the tear film washing over them...the muscles around the eyes begin__relax...

"And, since it is all connected...so too do the muscles in the face...and neck...and on down...so that it can be like an easy wave of relaxation extending in its own way from head to neck...and chest to abdomen... and legs to toes...

"And that can be happening now...or after a brief moment's hesitancy or resistance...and then letting go...."

> NOTE: If there is resistance, I need to name it and claim for it to be subsumed into the Linkage pattern. Thereafter, I can prescribe its disappearance.

"while on the inside...Gently breathing in [timed with Jane inhaling]... and out [timed with her exhalation] can allow you to discover the beginnings of a deepening sense of comfort and relaxation.... That's right...not too deep...just deep enough really relax..."

> NOTE: First, I DESCRIBE present conscious feelings—soothing tear film; then, I DESCRIBE verifiable preconscious experiences—facial relaxation and breathing; finally, I PRESCRIBE experiences—a wave of relaxation, a sense of increasing comfort and relaxation.

Sights

"And there are sights too…outside and inside…. So that even as the
EYES, JANE REMAIN CLOSED…there can be a soothing sense of light
and shadow on the back of the lids…while deeper inside you might
allow yourself to discover, some pleasant image from imagination
or recollection or combination…something you can safely enjoy…
observing the forms and figures…the colors and shades…all like in
a forgotten dream…just watching and enjoying…while forgetting,
without even knowing it…"

> NOTE: The same routine, using permissive language, only this time
> in the visual mode. Notice also how I am introducing the idea of
> forgetting, "like in a forgotten dream."

Sounds

"And, of course, there are sounds too…for example, the outside sound
of this voice can go with you wherever you, JANE GO INTO TRANCE …
and it can become whatever makes sense inside…like the sound of a
whispering breeze….

"And isn't it nice to know you don't even need to listen to every word,
because your unconscious WILL understand the meanings….

"And there are inside sounds, too…whether that's the sound of
breathing in [timed with inhalation] or breathing out [timed
with exhalation]…or, JANE EVEN DEEPER…the sounds of your own
thoughts…if you subvocalize, as some do…or of a musical memory…
or some other pleasant sound…."

> NOTE: Now, I am working in the acoustic mode. As I move from
> description to prescription, and from outside to inside, I am also
> seeding the idea that my voice can be part of a deep trance scene,
> like the wind I will soon be describing (below).

"So that there are just comfortable feelings...and sights that you can watch and enjoy...and the wonderful sounds as you, JANE BECOME EVEN MORE RELAX (sic)...MORE COMFORTABLE...

"It's a letting go.... As the old Hindus used to say: 'Like a salt doll dissolving safely in a warm sea of comfort'...no boundaries...just safe...just comfortable...watching...listening...in the place where the unconscious understands...and achieves... That's right."

> NOTE: I use this metaphor all the time as a trance deepening suggestion. It works well, so long as you remember to say "safely." As with all suggestions, observe for a response, and then ratify that response with an affirmation, "that's right."

Trance Utilization

There is no need to rush at this point. By now your patient should be exhibiting a paucity of non-prescribed behaviors. Let things settle. You needn't be concerned about "depth" of trance. I have witnessed the most extraordinary post-surgical results from patients who experience what would be deemed by many experts the lightest trance. What matters most is that there is evidence your patient is responding to your suggestions. When you suggest relaxation, inspect for signs of relaxation (e.g., shoulders lowering, respiratory rate slowing). When you suggest a visual image, look for their eyes to roll (generally upward). When you suggest smells, watch for the nostrils to flare. Take a few peaceful breaths, quietly, in unison with your patient.

Ego Strengthening

At this juncture, I often add a gentle line or two of acknowledgment and praise for the patient. Something like this:

"And as you allow yourself___settle even deeper...even safer...you might take a humble moment to privately acknowledge...after all you have been through...all you have worked to overcome...your true courage

and resourcefulness. Of course, there was some nervousness and very real concern…and yet, you summoned the fortitude…to find the right doctors and surgeons…to take the extra measures like learning to, JANE GO INTO TRANCE and enlist your unconscious…and let it protect you and rapidly return you to health…. A quiet breath to acknowledge yourself and recognize your strength and tenacity."

Therapeutic Suggestions

Then, I begin to offer the therapeutic suggestions we have both agreed to, including: no bleeding ("keep your blood"), no pain ("delightfully surprising comfort") and wound healing ("really rapid wound-healing"). I generally offer each suggestion three ways: directly (though usually somewhat softened), indirectly and metaphorically.

Of course, it is important to consistently maintain *Rapport* by delivering the messages with the rhythm of your patient's breathing. Similarly, Linkage is maintained by continuing to speak incontrovertibly (by using permissive language), naming it (e.g., any event that gains the patient's attention) and thereby claiming it, and finally, by LINKING your words to your patient's predictable future experiences (e.g., "delightfully surprising comfort"). Thus:

> *"Now many patients over the years, just like yourself, were nervous at first…until they realized…you can, JANE ALLOW YOURSELF TO RELAX AND REST…And that it can be as if there is a vast sunlit field… extending from end to end…a beautiful DRY FIELD …where you can just FEEL SAFE AND COMFORTABLE."*
>
> NOTE: I use "it can be as if" to introduce the metaphor of a dry field.
>
> *"And you can really begin to see it…that beautiful dry field…just dry… so that as the soft winds blow through…it whispers…[whispering close to the patient] 'keep your own blood…all your own blood inside… you don't need to lose a drop…just dry…dry as a bone…' And that's something the unconscious can understand…and WILL do…"*

> NOTE: The word "WILL" is controvertible...and so, it is **not** in the usual lexicon for Linkage. However, it has its place; and that place is when Authority is heightened, as it is here, and the need for emphasis is great.

"...even as this peaceful calm, which you can now, JANE EXPERIENCE THROUGH AND THROUGH, remains with you...as you drive to the hospital...as you walk through the doors...as you lie on the gurney... just calm and comfortable....

"So that any momentary nervousness you or others might have will be a trigger for even greater peacefulness and relaxation....

"And, of course, half a moment is a moment too...and half again..."

> NOTE: I know there is a chance the suggestion for calm and comfort might not fully manifest, so I anticipate the patient's breakthrough "momentary nervousness," name it and claim it (meaning, enfold it into the Linkage pattern) and prescribe its duration as an exponentially shrinking "moment."

"Just peaceful and calm...so that the entire operation is like a rediscovery of this vast dry field, warm...safe...dry...

"And in this dry field...as you discover some comfortable way to rest and really relax...you can allow yourself to see up ahead...somewhere in the near future...watching your own delightful surprise as you, JANE AWAKEN FROM SURGERY...PERFECTLY COMFORTABLE... DELIGHTFULLY SURPRISING COMFORT...surprising to both yourself and others around you.

*"Because your unconscious knows **it can forget to feel**...just as it forgets a dream...or a trance...or the back of an ankle...forgetting to feel... **just comfortable**.*

"So that when surprised doctors or nurses or friends ask, 'do you want pain medicine?' or 'how is your pain?' or 'can you rate your pain?'...

The word PAIN *is a trigger for the unconscious to make you* EVEN
MORE COMFORTABLE.*"*

> NOTE: My prediction about doctors, nurses or friends using the
> word "pain" describes the patient's inevitable future experience.
> This, in essence, extends the Linkage pattern into the future; and,
> since Patterns Persist, my next words can prescribe the patient's next
> future experience—whereby hearing the word "pain" triggers even
> more comfort. Notice also how the pearl-word "even" is used to
> presuppose an existing state of post-operative comfort.

"Because again, your conscious mind can **know** *what to move and not
move…so you can,* JANE FORGET TO FEEL…*because, you really do not
need to feel…"*

> NOTE: Nothing fancy. An indirect suggestion for comfort, "…you
> do not need to feel…"

*"And while you continue to rest and deeply relax…you can, Jane,
discover the broad sunlit path ahead…in the moments after surgery…
and the hours after…and the days after….And there you are…up
ahead, walking in perfect comfort and safety…your wounds healing
as if on their own clock…. Really rapid wound-healing…Which
is something the unconscious knows and* WILL *do…Really rapid
wound-healing…to the joyful astonishment of your doctor…really
rapid wound-healing…as you, Jane, walk on…day and night…just
comfortable."*

Trance Emergence

Just before I arouse a patient, I take them deeper. Naturally, many patients
are afraid to go "too deep," so I always make a point to connect "safer" with
"deeper." At this point Authority is often maximal, so direct suggestions are
more allowable.

Once the final suggestions are inculcated, I offer amnesia suggestions. Then,
I awaken the patient and immediately orient them to the outside world. As
Erickson pointed out, we have a lifetime pattern of waking, orienting to the

outside world and forgetting internal goings-on (e.g., our dreams). Patterns Persist.

> *"And now you can take a deep breath and, as you exhale…Jane, allow yourself__go even deeper…into the restful silences…into the deeper, safer parts of the unconscious…where dreams are made and… forgotten.*

> *"And this trance can be like a forgotten dream where only the unconscious remembers: keep your blood…delightfully surprising comfort…really-rapid-wound-healing…*

> *"While you discover something so beautiful…something you just watch and marvel at…so beautiful…like a butterfly's wings or a rainbow or a gorgeous smile…something that you really can remember…while you forget the rest…"*

>> NOTE: I have found it useful to offer something the patient can remember. As you'll see, I use that image almost immediately upon emergence.

> *"Even as you find some pleasant, happy way to let your conscious mind wake up refreshed and alert in the here and…NOW."*

All patients awaken differently: some slow, some fast; some animated, some relatively still. The key, as always, is to observe for arousal behaviors ("Uh-huh"), ratify those behaviors ("…that's right") and augment them with encouraging suggestions ("…all the way awake").

> *Patient: Ahh…*

> *You: That's right…all the way awake…refreshed and alert….Hi there.*

>> NOTE: When Erickson was asked why, when a patient first woke, he routinely said "Howdy," he replied: "It's the language of consciousness."

> *Patient: (Rubbing their eyes.)*

You: Remember where you parked your car?

> NOTE: This swiftly returns them to their external reality.

Patient: Um…yeah.

You: And before you forget everything…what was that beautiful thing?

Patient: Beautiful thing? Oh, yes, it was a rainbow. I remembered it from Maui.

You: Wonderful. And I suppose there are many more beautiful memories ahead. Now, will you call me and let me know how well things go tomorrow?

Patient: I certainly will.

You: And don't be opposed to surprising yourself.

Patient: Oh, I won't. Thank you.

Summing Up

The basic elements in this transcript for presurgical hypnosis are simple. First, seed the ideas and agree on shared goals. Then, induce a trance using Linkage and *Rapport* (and your Authority) to create a unique, comfortable and unfamiliar experience for the patient. During that experience (which enhances your Authority), offer the therapeutic suggestions directly, indirectly and metaphorically. Then, suggest "conscious forgetting" and unconscious DOING. Finally, awaken the patient while remaining cognizant of your continuing influence over events.

I have put some flavor and flourish into this dialogue, so you can see how all the refinements we've been discussing can come together. But remember the lessons of placebo: Even if the preceding suggestions were offered straight-up from an unartful Authority, roughly a third of patients would likely respond with favorable outcomes. Take heart in knowing this. Then, practice and enjoy.

HEALING: BEYOND PILLS & POTIONS

"The nature and force of a disease must be discovered by their cause not by their symptoms...for we must not merely extinguish the smoke of the fire but the fire itself."

—Paracelsus, 16th century

Chapter 12:
STRATEGIES FOR CURE

WE NOW HAVE ALL THE REQUISITE SKILLS to go for what I call "deep cures." We understand that virtually all disease is multifactorial, and that both material and mental causes can contribute to the penetration of Host Defenses and manifest as Signs and Symptoms. In modern times, traditional reductionist science has been brilliant in curtailing the physical effects of material causes, and we can all be thankful for its continuing progress. But what happens when only the material causes of an ailment have been addressed? Isn't it reasonable to suspect that unchallenged noetic causes, when they exist, sustain their attack? And if so, shouldn't we expect to discover patient after patient suffering one disease after another, notwithstanding one reductionist "cure" after another?

Blunt Beginnings and Endless Endings

In fact, isn't that what we do see? That is precisely what my Family Practice patient, Carol, was exhibiting for the three years I managed her care. Her real diagnosis, in my present view, was not the extended list of infections, conditions and syndromes reported in her three-inch-thick chart. Her real diagnosis was, "impaired Host Defenses, secondary to unknown (probably noetic) causes." Had I known how to take a more thorough history, had I understood the true nature of symptom formation, had I developed the skills to address the various contributing causes of Carol's illnesses—perhaps I could have helped her more. After all, our Expanded Causal Model implies that when a sufficient number of causes are deactivated, Host Defenses revive and Health is restored. Returning to our gyroscope metaphor, it is as if the central spin is once again revved, rendering minor and even major perturbations incapable of "toppling the top."

Remember Michael, the 129lb patient in Chapter 8 who was dying from acute graft versus host disease? His "causes" manifested first as a highly aggressive lymphoma, refractory to traditional agents. Ultimately, Michael required massive chemotherapy to obliterate the tumor and allow for bone marrow transplantation. Yet, no sooner did the graft "take," then he was stricken with graft versus host disease, and after that, with a rampant CMV (a virus) infection. Despite the full armamentarium of modern medicines, Michael continued to manifest disease after disease. In other words, Michael's hydra-headed presentation fit the profile of a patient with unaddressed Zone I-Causes.

It was clear, in Michael's case, that the material causes of his disease were properly treated with conventional medications. But, as you will recall, I suspected three common noetic causes that were unaddressed: namely, **Guilt** (over not having grieved his father's passing "properly"), a **Dangerous Identification** (with his "a patient all his life" father, who had died at Michael's exact age) and **Retreat into Illness** (in hopes of drawing back his estranged girlfriend). I also suspected there might be other unknown noetic causes lurking.

Michael's case provides an instructive test of our new conception of Health and Healing—of mind mattering, of the tendential nature of symptom formation and the curative potential of well-wrought suggestions. So, let's now turn to the details I promised back in Chapter 8—specifically, how to treat Michael's persistent noetic causes so as to bring about a lasting cure.

What follows is the distilled essence of my approach, which spanned several sessions. As you already know, it worked. Michael remains, more than 10 years later, disease-free, "happy and engaged in life." So, too, are the numerous other patients I have treated using the methods outlined below: patients diagnosed with refractory lung cancer, advanced heart disease, pervasive autoimmune disease, crippling arthritis and more, including dense psychopathy. As effective as these methods have been, I have no doubt (and great hope) that in the future, even better and more effective protocols will be innovated and shared by practitioners of the Exquisite Art.

I. Defusing the Guilt Bomb

Remember from our earlier discussion that guilt often entails both shame and suffering. As Lucretius observed, "The guilty mind is its own torturer." This concept is not inherent in the human psyche; it must be learned. Perhaps not surprisingly, discovering the original source of one's guilt concept can be instrumental in effecting a cure: particularly since working within the fixed framework of one's entrenched ideas is easier than attempting to uproot those ideas. In this regard, the key question to ask during Information Gathering is not "what religion are you?" but rather, "what religion did you grow up in?" For example, if the answer is Catholicism, the caregiver understands that the concepts of absolution and divine forgiveness exist within the system. This knowledge can have great utility.

Once the source of the guilt concept is understood, and the inciting event of the patient's guilt is gleaned from their history, it is time to formulate therapeutic suggestions and offer them effectively. Below are three approaches, all of which I used in Michael's case:

A. Reframing the Offense

Numerous books and articles have been written using the term "reframing" to indicate a variety of therapeutic methods. To be clear, what I mean by reframing is the replacement of one frame or perspective through which a given event is viewed with another frame or perspective through which that same event can be viewed, albeit differently.

Thus, Michael's reaction to his father's death was perceived by Michael, throughout his life, from a 13-year old's perspective, following the imputation of wrongdoing by his mother. An adult might have discounted her distracted accusations, but not her young child: In essence, Michael had committed the sin of improper grieving and deserved to be shamed and punished.

Useful understandings for reframing Michael's reaction are:

1. Everyone grieves differently. There is no right way.
2. Denial often strikes people immediately upon learning of a death, only to relent after sufficient time has passed. (Michael—who went by "Mikey" in those days— did break down and cry profusely about two weeks after his father's passing.)
3. All kids want to be accepted, to be "cool." Having a brain-injured dad set Michael apart and was embarrassing. He was too young to know how to handle the challenge differently. In other words, Michael's reaction was normal for a child his age.

This is the "frame" of a sensible adult—the necessary substitute for Michael's persisting childhood perspective. In the transcript below, we will see how that substitution is implemented.

B. Restructuring the Punishment

Two principles warrant consideration when looking for leverage against guilt-induced symptoms: justice and purpose. Justice, within most belief systems, requires that the punishment fit the crime: "an eye for an eye." Purpose implies that the punishment should teach the sufferer a lesson.

I often "seed" both of these ideas well before trance induction, observing the patient closely for signs of agreement or disagreement. In Michael's case, for example, it was agreed early on that a child failing to grieve as expected is not a "mortal sin." The implication is that death would, therefore, be an unjust punishment for his relatively minor infraction. Further, Michael accepted that the ideal punishment—in the abstract—is one that, fulfilling its purpose, forever reminds the "sinner" what not to do.

"I am reminded," I tell Michael, as if casually recollecting, "of W. C. Fields' comment when, a noose around his neck, the hangman asked if he had any last words. 'This is going to be a great lesson to me,' he quipped."

> NOTE: This is an ironic metaphor conveying the notion, Death is a Poor Teacher.

Next, I introduced the idea that "knowledge of sin is often the worst punishment." First, I suggested to Michael: "Wouldn't most children rather have one slap on the wrist, and have it done than be brow-beaten and scolded every day for a year?" Then, I went on to explain that the **knowledge of a wrongdoing is a constant punishment**: "Just knowing you hurt someone you love, for example, is forever a punishing thought."

Thus, it became established in what seemed like casual talk, that:

1. justice would be better served by meting out a non-lethal punishment, and
2. the purpose of that punishment would be better fulfilled by substituting a sustained, unforgettable knowledge of the wrongdoing for actual physical symptoms.

Recall, I had also speculated that there might be another purpose of the punishment—namely, to teach Michael what his invalid father had suffered.

In this regard, I added: "But let me ask you this, if the purpose of all this was somehow to have you experience suffering, have you learned that lesson?"

Michael teared up, "Have I ever...," he said.

*"Well, as a wiser man than me once said," I again offer casually, "if you can have a piece of an experience, you can have it all. Which I guess means that if you can experience a period of real suffering, then you can **Michael truly understand** what your father's lifetime of suffering must have been like."*

NOTE: This suggestion, which I use often and in a variety of ways, allows Michael to forgo a lifetime of suffering, by virtue of a simple act of sympathetic imagination. In essence I am suggesting that the punishment he is currently suffering has already fulfilled its purpose.

C. Forgiving the Offense

Forgiveness can come from three sources—oneself, the one offended and the divine power. I cover all three, beginning with oneself. As you'll see in the script below, I lace self-forgiveness into the reframing portion of work. Here I am often reminded of Erickson's famous Monde case, in which he suggests to a guilt-ridden 30-year-old Monde that she look back (in trance) at her child-self playing mischievously: "And a child that age," Erickson offers gently, "can never do anything that is really very bad, can they?" (Notice the tag-question.)

I then move to the offended party:

> *"Your mother, at the height of her own overwhelming grief, could not have understood her little boy's denial—his immediate need to block the pain. Nor could she have understood, in those painful moments, the normal relief from 'being different' that any 13-year-old would have felt.... A young boy with normal emotions...whom she loves and...now, of course, most certainly forgives."*

Last there is the divine power, the final arbiter, who alone can declare: "You have suffered enough." Imagine telling a patient, no matter what your Authority, that God told you this. It is simply not credible. Not effective. And yet, if you exercise care and patience in trance induction and deepening, once the patient is sufficiently deep and capable of amnesia, you can offer this:

> *"It is as if from the deepest deep...from directions far and wide...the omniscient voice that has never lied...that can only speak the deepest truth...declares...[long pause] Michael, you have suffered enough... you have suffered enough."*

In such cases, it is as if the patient experiences "the voice" directly. Done right, this singular suggestion can have the most profound curative effect on guilt-engendered disease.

Trance Tips

Guilt arises from a deep source and therefore is often best addressed from a position of maximal Authority. In many cases, though not always (recall the new mother with pelvic pain, Chapter 5), this means having the patient in hypnotic trance. Method matters here. Accordingly, once trance is induced, I "deepen" it by gradually evoking behaviors perceived by the patient to be more and more non-normal and non-voluntary. Each step enhances my Authority, making my next suggestions ever more likely to actualize.

The non-voluntary nature of prescribed behaviors is achieved by ascribing their source not to "YOU" the patient, but rather to "the unconscious" or "It," which operates outside of "You." Of course, the motive force driving the idea of unconscious causation is the momentum imparted by the three dominant hypnotic patterns—namely, Authority, *Rapport* and Linkage.

As to the non-ordinary behaviors, I suggest "the unconscious" create them in increments, progressing generally from one to the next as follows:

> 1. "…a certain degree of pleasant tingling…or warmth…somewhere
> on the body…And you can, Michael really feel that, can't you?"
> (Then, OBSERVE >> RATIFY >> AUGMENT.)
> 2. "…a particular amount of pleasant heaviness…which you might
> begin to feel…in one foot or the other…or somewhere there-
> abouts…" (Same reinforcing sequence.)
> 3. "…and the hand can begin to feel lighter and lighter…even as
> the unconscious first decides which hand…and then, as if breath by
> breath (said on inhalations) …lighter and lighter…it begins to lift…
> to float…just floating." (Thus inducing hand levitation and catalepsy,
> "That's right…even higher.")

4. And finally, with the hand afloat, I suggest that "…boundaries dissolve…like a salt doll dissolving safely in a warm sea of comfort… just letting go…."

Of course, during this entire process of trance deepening, I carefully maintain *Rapport* and Linkage. I should note that hypnosis textbooks are replete with methods for trance deepening, and many of these methods (though they may err on the theory side) are quite effective. Whatever your technique, the deeper the trance the more likely you often are to defuse your patient's guilt.

Trance Script

Now, let's look at the therapeutic suggestions that flow from the foregoing considerations. While I will compress this into a single brief transcript, please understand that it may take two or three sessions to present and repeat all that follows:

Let's assume trance has been induced, using the technique from the previous chapter, and that deepening measures are complete.

> "*…And isn't it nice to, Michael discover that you can be **here** in a safe and comfortable trance, **just watching your** younger self, 'Mikey,' over there…*"

>> NOTE: I direct my voice "here" toward the patient, Michael, when speaking to him; and "over there" toward the patient's younger self, "Mikey," when referring to him.

> "*…first hearing the news of his father's death…then, feeling a natural sense of relief…a 13-year-old's natural sense of relief…at no longer having to be different…*

> "*…even as unconscious Denial blocks young Mikey's true sorrow…his deep sorrow over a father's passing…something a 13-year-old is not yet ready to fully grasp…*

> "*…any more than he can fully understand his mother's blind grief… her turning on him for just a moment…because, of course, just*

watching her…there was nowhere else for her to turn…in her crushing grief…And it's all so clear to see…

"*…A young boy being a normal 13-year-old. A mother being a grieving wife…People being their true selves…doing their very best in a sad, sad moment…*

"*…And it's okay to wish little Mikey had done better…Because he did go on to learn…to have a whole lifetime of compassion…and caring… and giving to others…*

"*…And, of course, his mother whose grief would lessen with time… forgives him now…And here in a pleasant deepening trance, you can, Michael, forgive young Mikey, too…and really feel that love and forgiveness for him.…Acting like a young boy when he was a young boy…*

"*It's like a gentle rain washing all the dust and dirt off a long-parked car—stuff that does not need to be there anymore…that even your unconscious knows it can* LET GO.…

"*Because **just knowing** what happened is punishment enough…and you will always remember that…and learn from it…*

"*It's like an unfixed dent on that car, that always reminds you…and **just knowing is punishment enough**…*

"*Now, you can Michael go even deeper…just safely letting go…as if into the deep, wide silences of trance…wherefrom there comes a hallowed voice…a voice as if from all sides…omniscient…a voice that can only speak the truth…[A long pause here, building response potential. Breathing in sync with the patient.]*

"*And it proclaims…Michael, you have suffered enough.…And even as it speaks you can feel the truth in every atom…in every cell…Michael, you have suffered enough.*"

II. Dangerous Identifications

The helpless and dependent child, in order to survive, must identify with The One least uncertain. This identification with the Authority has a profound effect on present and future attributes and behaviors. The young child, immersed in the "My Reality (i.e., the Authority) = Your Reality" (i.e., the child) pattern, unconsciously absorbs how to perceive and navigate the world, how to relate to other people including oneself, how to behave as a parent toward children and spouse, to react to challenges, to set and achieve goals—a whole constellation of defining traits and activities that compel, in broad strokes, the course of an individual's life.

This is why people tend to marry (in their first marriage, at least) someone like their opposite-sex parent (e.g., in heterosexual marriages) and "become their parents" once their children are born. This is why people often love or hate themselves (and others) in the same manner as their original Authority figure; and why they affiliate as their original Authority figure did, religiously and politically…and so on.

In my view, far too much has been made of psychodynamic interpretations of behavior, and even of genetics, and far too little of the imitative propensity.

In Michael's case, identification with his patient-father almost certainly played a role in the etiology of his disease. This was reconfirmed one day after Michael's recovery when I overheard him describe to others what he believed had been the source of his cure: "I stopped being a patient," he said. This struck me as particularly revelatory since during our first interview Michael had described his father as "always a patient." It's easy to conceive how Michael's paternal-identification (with a man who suffered much and ultimately died from his illness) conspired with the other two noetic causes— guilt and the wish to retreat into illness—to generate one punishing illness after another.

The question is, how does one sever all or part of these early childhood identifications when they are suspected of contributing to disease?

I generally begin by seeding the idea that the childhood bonds can be broken without dishonoring the parent—and that, in fact, dissolving those bonds is the best way to attain personal growth and an adult loving relationship with that Authority figure.

> *"You know, Michael…some scientists think we can never be closer to anyone in life than we are to our mother, in utero, before the cord was cut. And yet, if you think about it…while that may be true for a fetus…closeness and love and honor are very different for an adult.*
>
> *"Because, when we are tied to someone as adults…there is often some hidden resentment…that prevents us from seeing who they really are…who we really are…*
>
> *"For example, it's only when YOU TRULY CUT THE CORD…that you can…Michael, see who your parents truly are…and love them for that…in a new, independent way.*
>
> *"And, you can also see who you really are…and that you have your own independent way of being your best you.*
>
> *"Because we really don't need to be bound to someone we truly love. You can, MICHAEL CUT THE CORD and love them for all their faults and foibles…for all their gifts and grace…and you **honor** them best with that kind of adult love and understanding."*

>> NOTE: In the Judeo-Christian tradition, the young child is taught to "Honor thy father and thy mother." (In many systems, it is a potentially guilt-inducing "sin" to do otherwise.) Early on, this can only mean "Obey thy father and thy mother." An adult understanding of "honor" is generally acquired much later, if ever.
>>
>> Therefore, the suggestion above is liberating: It is okay to "cut the cord." You honor your parents best, not through obedience or umbilical dependency, but rather through a freely chosen love—one based on gratitude and unforced feelings of affection.
>>
>> In Michael's case, this essentially permits him NOT to "be a patient" (as his father was), while still honoring his father.

I then proceed to reframe the patient's conception of the Authority figure. This can be done both while the patient is awake and, later, in trance. Remember, the young child bonds with the Authority as he or she perceives that Authority. But childhood impressions are almost never entirely accurate or complete; there is almost always another perspective. In Michael's case, for example, he perceived his father to be "a patient all his life." A victim. And yet, there is certainly another perspective far more conducive to Michael's health:

> *"And, of course, a young boy almost never sees as clearly as his adult-self will see…*
>
> *"Imagine, for example, your father over there in his chair…happy and peaceful…his wife, your mother, by his side…having survived the war…having survived the blast…having survived the injury…He was a patient, yes…but beyond that…as your adult eyes can now see… he was a survivor…..A true survivor."*

Finally, I offer the central suggestion, which is, essentially, a combination of the two tactics above—namely, you can sever your childhood ties to your childhood Authority figure and, nonetheless, honor that Authority by being your best. In Michael's case: "Michael, you no longer need to be 'a patient.' You can now choose to be a survivor." I usually offer these deeply transformative ideas in trance, as metaphorical suggestions:

> *"It is as if we are all born on a comfortable raft, slowly being drawn down the river by its powerful current…sleeping…resting… unaware of the current into which we are born. Time passes…and gradually a young boy begins to sense the river…the pull of the current…and for a while it may seem alright…*
>
> *"It is only later when the waters roughen…and later still when the roar of the approaching waterfall can be heard…that the boy, who is now a man…becomes anxious…and fearful…*

"And it is at this moment…that the man becomes aware…and realizes the danger of the current…the current he has been so PATIENT *in…and decides to* MICHAEL, STOP BEING A PATIENT *and swim… swim to where* YOU CHOOSE *to be."*

> NOTE: The phonologic ambiguity between being PATIENT and being A PATIENT, which I am playing on to Michael's advantage. Also, the underscored suggestion to STOP BEING A PATIENT.

"And so, he sets his sights on his destination…to SURVIVE…

"Of course, it isn't easy at first…the current is strong…but you fight it with conscious resolve to survive…you, Michael, stay aware… consciously at times…and unconsciously always… and discover you too are strong.…And soon you are on the shore…and clambering up the high embankment…and out onto the vast sunlit plane of opportunities…and you realize…somewhere deep inside… YOU ARE A SURVIVOR…MICHAEL, YOU ARE A SURVIVOR…

"And as you, Michael, bask in your robust health…you look back and discover…as they all discover…that the enormous river, the deep ravine, the gorge from which you climbed…it is but a tiny crack…a small fissure…in the vast field of joy and health and choice…that remains open to you now."

This, of course, is a classic metaphor for leaving the parental "current" and setting one's own direction, sustaining the struggle consciously and unconsciously, and emerging triumphant. In its many variations, I have found it immensely useful. For, to one degree or another, we are all in that current until we choose otherwise.

III. Retreat into Illness

This is one of the most common noetic causes of illness in advanced cultures. As we discussed in Chapter 7, it is learned—I dare say "conditioned"—in childhood and often recurs reflexively. It is a dangerous pattern, especially when recklessly evoked with the phrase "…no matter what," as when a patient mutters: "I've got to get out of this situation, NO MATTER WHAT."

Recall the frustrated Staff Physician listed in Chapter 2 who, disappointed with hospital understaffing, strongly affirmed to himself: "I've got to get out of this job, no matter what." Twenty-seven hours later, he was battling one of the most virulent bacterial infections known to humankind—meningococcemia. It can kill in just four hours.

As the penicillin and Rocephin™ flooded his veins, he could be heard reciting T.S. Elliot's famous refrain: "That is not what I meant, at all. That is not what I meant, at all.…"

P.S. Thanks to an early self-diagnosis, he lived. Lesson learned.

In Chapter 2, we also discussed the one promising aspect of this otherwise treacherous coping mechanism, namely: "If the door can swing one way toward sickness, it can swing the other way toward health." If a patient's unconscious can make them sick, it can also make them well. I **seed** this idea during what most often seems like casual conversation.

Michael (in response to my query, "Why now?"): I don't know. I suppose if I had to guess, I might say some part of me might have thought that maybe being sick would lure my girlfriend back…I guess.

Me: And, of course, didn't we all do something like that when we were young and had limited options? Most kids, for instance, discover that to gain someone's attention or avoid humiliation at school, they can generate a sore throat, or tummy ache or some other symptom…

Michael: Sure, I mean, I did that…

Me: And did you ever think about what happened once the attention was gained or after the undesirable event passed? Did you stay sick, or get worse?

Michael: No, I got well.

Me: Because the same unconscious part that actualized your wish to be sick heard your new wish to be well, and IT MAKES YOU WELL. If the door can swing one way toward illness, it certainly WILL swing the other way toward health. (This is done, of course, with proper hand gesturing.)

Michael: Un-huh.

Later, I offer Michael the following suggestions, which promote the gracious exchange of childhood habits for healthy adult choices.

"It's like when you were very young, and first learned to crawl…and crawling was your only means of locomotion. For a time, if you wanted to go somewhere, that was your only choice.

"Of course, as you got older, your choices expanded…. Soon, you learned to walk, and skip, and run…to ride a bicycle…eventually to drive a car or take an airplane. A vast world of adult choices opened up…

"And, you can still crawl if you choose…if it is a really tight space…but the choice is yours…

"And isn't that how things so often are? In childhood, we really do have limited choices…whereas as adults…your choices are so many….

"And so, in childhood, our unconscious problem-solver often becomes a symptom-maker…a tummy ache or sore throat solves the problem of the day…. What other choices did it have…?

"And yet, in adulthood—a time when symptoms become less desirable…when you really do not need to have a symptom—the same predicament can be solved in so many different ways.

"Wanting a loved one's attention, for instance, prompts a child to cry… whereas an adult can have a conversation…or write a poem…or ask

what's wrong.…An adult can even reconsider.… Is she really right for me?…or, should I make some constructive changes in myself and find someone more suited to me?

*"A host of choices for **the unconscious** problem-solver to choose from…as **it** operates on an important new principle…a law of sorts, to guide and protect you… ONLY HEALTHY SOLUTIONS.…*

*"So that each time a problem is raised, **the unconscious** will understand, a thought or an action is okay…but never a symptom… ONLY HEALTHY SOLUTIONS…*

*"The new governing principle of **the unconscious**…kept as deep as your firmest beliefs…as deep as your knowledge of who you are and where you came from…deep where your very name is kept… ONLY HEALTHY SOLUTIONS…*

*"As **it** discovers…as if with the utmost deep delight…the profound joy of choosing to… MICHAEL, BECOMING A HEALTHY SURVIVOR…[long pause].*

"That's right…and as this new governing principle sinks deeply, deeply in… ONLY HEALTHY SOLUTIONS…you can, Michael, take all the time you need in the next 2 to 3 minutes…to wake up…as A HEALTHY SURVIVOR." (Thus, concluding with a double bind.)

Of course, if your patient could do this consciously, chances are they would have done so. Therefore, the Artful Caregiver uses his or her skills to enlist a dissociated agency ("IT," "the unconscious") that operates outside of conscious volition to do the work. And as we now know, the driving forces behind that agency are the persisting patterns of Authority, *Rapport* and Linkage.

When thinking about how to offer therapeutic suggestions, remember this: There is only one way to do it wrong, and that is to ignore the "cause" and fail to address it. The Placebo Effect teaches us that even with a modicum of Authority, our suggestions often actualize. Therefore, however elegantly or inelegantly we present these salutary ideas—so long as we use the Exquisite Art to the best of our present ability—our patients will likely have an improved outcome. Not always, perhaps, but often.

IV. Curses

Michael did not disclose the casting of any curses (i.e., negative suggestions) from the medical establishment. But there is one curse so prevalent today that I elected to address it, just in case. It is the notion that genes ineluctably determine one's fate.

This notion ignores the fact of "variable penetration" and the causal implications of this well-established phenomenon. In a nutshell, the term refers to the fact that genes "penetrate" to phenotypic expression variably—manifesting as a full-blown expression of the underlying gene in one person, partial expression in another and no expression whatsoever in yet another. Moreover, this can vary within the individual over time. The implication, of course, is that there are numerous factors in addition to genetics (so-called epigenetics) that determine the expression or suppression of such genes.

What I wanted to do in Michael's case was address whatever negative suggestions might have been insinuated by his various doctors concerning the "inevitable expression" of his mutation. This was done both with waking suggestion and in trance:

> *"At some point, perhaps sooner rather than later, you can discover the truth of what so many of the most advanced minds in human genetics are now proclaiming...*
>
> *"...namely, 'Genetics is not Destiny'... 'Genetics is not Destiny'...*
>
> *"...which means...not all genes express themselves...some stay quiet... others return to the quiescence after a while...especially...*
>
> *"As the unconscious understands...ONLY HEALTHY SOLUTIONS... Only Healthy Solutions."*

V. Unknown Causes

I generally assume that the noetic causes I have surmised are not the only ones contributing to a patient's illness. This may or may not be true. But since the approach to dealing with unknown noetic causes is benign, there is no harm in adding these additional salutary suggestions to the mix.

In this regard, we have already addressed the insertion of the "ONLY HEALTHY SOLUTIONS" proviso into the Zone III-Principle of Parsimony. Recall, the basic function of this Principle is to fulfill as many Zone I-Causes as possible with a minimum number of solutions (preferably one), regardless of whether those solutions are healthy or not. Our treatment of the Retreat into Illness wish modified this operating principle to preclude all illnesses from consideration as possible solutions: "ONLY HEALTHY SOLUTIONS."

For cancer patients, like Michael, I often tweak this proviso by calling for "ONLY HEALTHY CELLS." I tend to insert this idea as deeply as possible, with as much Authority as possible, during hypnotic trance. Additionally, I will often offer it as an affirmation, "Say ONLY HEALTHY CELLS, not 9 times, nor 11 times, but exactly 10 times, whenever the idea of cancer comes to mind. At first, of course, that will be fairly frequent. But with time, as the tumor shrinks, the idea will occur to you less and less frequently…and eventually, not at all." (NOTE: By now, I am sure you understand the nuances of this indirect suggestion for a cure.)

In this connection, people often ask: "Well, that's all well and good. But what about giving a clear biologic image of the immune system destroying the tumor? Isn't that even better?" This is a worthy question, so let's consider its origins and then ponder the answer.

Beginning in the 1970s with Dr. O. Carl Simonton and his wife, people began to believe that by using imagery analogous to the biological entities involved in immunity, patients could facilitate cancer regressions and cures.

A Pacman gobbling up "ghosts," for example, was thought to be sufficiently analogous to killer T-cells devouring cancer cells to direct cellular immunity against an existing tumor. The broad benefit of this approach, in addition to resulting in some remarkable outcomes, was that in some circles it elevated Noetic Medicine to a position of credibility. At the time, no small feat. However, one detriment was that implicit in this kind of thinking (though I do not ascribe this to the Simontons) was the notion that the more accurate the imagery—meaning, the more precisely it depicts the actual biologic entities and processes involved (e.g., cells, proteins, molecules)—the more beneficial it will be. I suppose this is possible. Fortunately, it is an empirical question that one day, perhaps noetic scientists will answer.

In the meantime, it is important that the details of the Simontons' approach not distract us from the underlying structure of that approach—a structure of doubtless efficacy, in and of itself. Recall from our earlier discussions, the **Placebo Effect is an Authority-driven, (non-trance) hypnotic response to the implicit suggestion "If you do x, then y—the prescribed effect will occur,"** provided that "x" is:

1. credible upon presentation;
2. somewhat difficult to achieve but achievable;
3. credible upon completion.

The Therapeutic Ritual the Simontons devised complies perfectly with these requirements:

1. The patient must first go to a hallowed place of science, meet with a physician bedecked in the trappings (white coat, stethoscope, diploma) of Authority, and receive complex instructions regarding an unusual mental exercise that must be performed in a certain way with a specified frequency. At the outset, (x) is credible; so, Authority is undiminished.

2. Getting to the physician/Authority took effort—an appointment had to be made, schedules arranged, transportation obtained. Then, further effort

was necessary to generate the requisite mental imagery and perform the exercise as specified. All somewhat difficult to achieve, but achievable. So far, nothing to discredit the Authority in any way.

3. The exercise itself does not dissuade the patient of its potential efficacy. It isn't too easy, too ordinary, too outlandish; in fact, it remains entirely credible upon completion.

In other words, the prerequisites for a successful Therapeutic Ritual are met perfectly by the Simonton ritual, and so the mighty forces behind the Placebo Effect (the "doctor within") are summoned.

Again, it may be that the more accurate the imagery, the more effective the suggestion. But I doubt it. After all, our current scientific explanations are merely the therapeutic metaphors of the day. Regardless of how accurate they may seem to us, one hundred years from now, they will have changed significantly. And yet, the present explanations work. Just as the stories told by sages work. Just as the many therapeutic metaphors I have referenced work. What matters, I would argue, is not the accuracy of the symbols, but rather their dynamic relationships. So long as the imagery does not undermine Authority, it will evoke a Placebo Effect.

Instead of focusing on (x), the "antecedent" in the Generic Placebo Suggestion, let me suggest we focus on (y), the "consequent." Consider this:

> *I am the first to go. Before me stretches 10m of red-hot oak coals. My shoes and socks have been cast off, my pants rolled up.*
>
> *Before I walk across the 1000 °F bed of coals, I repeat my self-suggestion: "My unconscious will do whatever it needs to do to protect me." I do not say: "My unconscious will gush sweat from my soles, or my unconscious will decrease the thermal conductivity of my feet."*
>
> *Then, I look up and think "cool moss," while plodding over the embers.*
>
> *Seconds later, I step out of the pit unscathed. Not so much as a blister.*

*My unconscious has done as directed: "...whatever **it** needs to do to protect me."*

> NOTE: The implicit placebo suggestion leading up to the firewalk was, "If (x) you roll your eyes up and think 'Cool moss,' then (y) your unconscious will do whatever is necessary to protect you."

In this connection, I often ask my patients (as I did with Michael) to stand and walk to the door. Once they have done that, I ask them to turn around and imagine a fine line on the floor, extending from where they now stand to their chair. I then say, "Now, walk back to your chair, being certain that with each step your second toe lands precisely on that fine line." Of course, it is much more difficult to walk back focused on each individual step than it was to walk away focused only on the goal.

Back to Michael:

> *Me: I consider these little demonstrations nontrivial because they show us the world of the mind in a microcosm.*
>
> *Michael: How so?*
>
> *Me: When you focused your conscious mind on the goal, your unconscious understood the mission and carried it out. You didn't need to focus on each swing of the leg, strike of the heel, lift of the knee. The unconscious did whatever it needed to do to get you to your chosen destination.*
>
> *Michael: I see. Very interesting.*
>
> *Me: So, what do you see yourself doing when you are well?*
>
> *Michael: You mean if I get over this?*
>
> *Me: I mean, where shall we direct **the unconscious** to take you? After all, **it** is flying the plane.*
>
> *Michael: I want to be on a beach in Hawaii, healthy and happy.*

Me: So, as you focus on that goal, the unconscious—which we will enlist fully in trance—will do whatever it needs to do to get you there. Because that, as we have just demonstrated, is how it works.

Again, since the implicit structure of the patient/caregiver encounter entails the Generic Placebo Suggestion, what matters most is (y) the "consequent"—the result. So long as (x) meets the criteria we have discussed, it will suffice. What matters most is the effect produced by fulfillment of the suggestion. This simple technique strengthens Host Defenses against whatever unknown causes might be active: "The unconscious will do whatever it needs to do..." to defeat them.

A Word About "Stress"

You will, perhaps, notice I did not list "stress" among the common noetic causes of illness. This is because the way this word is bandied about today, I don't know what it means. Even Dr. Hans Selye—renowned for his work on the general physiological response to certain stresses—became vexed with the abuse and nebulosity of the word. In response, he abandoned the term in favor of "stressor," for which he designated physical, chemical and psychological subcategories.

As regards psychological causes, I work to reduce them to their underlying **wishes,** because it is through **the volitional system,** especially when potentiated by the sympathetic nervous system, that dull ideas become noetic javelins hurled at Host Defenses. In cases of guilt-engendered illness, for example, there is always the wish to be punished. It takes very little perspicacity to glimpse the nature of the punishment required: one has only to look at the disease and its effects as the wish-fulfilled. In Michael's case, for example, the required punishment was to suffer and die at the age his father died. Similarly, Retreat into Illness generally contains an ill-framed generic wish to "get out of something." In such cases, the "symptom-maker/problem-solver" (i.e., Zones III-VI) will generally produce the most economic symptom by selecting one that satisfies the greatest number of importuning Zone 1-Causes.

Dangerous Identifications, I should note, are different. Here, an atavistic imitation principle operates, one prior to volition. There is no underlying wish, no psychodynamic interpretation. There is only monkey see, monkey do. But even here, knowing the Authority with whom your patient has identified, and the characteristics or behaviors your patient is taking on through imitation, provides you with the necessary information to fashion effective therapeutic suggestions.

To forego these queries and attribute disease simply to "stress" is, in my view, little more than a lazy nod to the possibility of psychological causes. Not that, in the effort to reduce "stress," changing one's external environment and adopting a sense of humor about one's predicament isn't salutary. It is. Such measures generally bolster Host Defenses. But the reason your patient has not already taken those measures, and frequently ignores your pleadings to do so, is often because of specific noetic causes like the ones we have been discussing. Knowing those causes allows you to target their eradication directly.

A Word About Affirmation

Affirmation—the so-called Power of Positive Thinking—certainly has its place in self-direction and self-healing. Many authors have written eloquently on this topic, urging strong, repetitive, conscious insistence on a goal. It is likely, especially when unopposed by countervailing noetic forces, these conscious directives have an effect: essentially, fortifying Host Defenses—revving, as it were, the gyro's central spin. In and of itself, Affirmation is a subject worthy of study and elaboration.

However, countervailing forces often exist; ambivalence is a common human condition. A self-engendered "Only Healthy Cells" affirmation, from a patient with cancer, might very well be opposed by malignant unconscious influences pressing for expression. And my experience is that when such noetic forces exist, simple affirmations are often not enough. Virtually all of the patients discussed so far came to me with positive attitudes, and many had mantras of their own. Yet, as we have seen, unattended noetic forces pressed on, eventuating in Endless Endings despite targeted remedies and positive thinking.

Simply put: **It takes more than positive, conscious thinking to eradicate negative unconscious thoughts.**

Fortunately, the Exquisite Art provides caregivers with various means of uprooting or subverting unconscious noetic influences. We have learned, for example, that Authority can sometimes overpower such influences by commanding the forces of health and healing—forestalling pain, preventing bleeding, relaxing airways—even rectifying aberrant heart rhythms. Further, we have learned how Indirection and other elements of the Art enable us to bypass resistances (i.e., the countervailing forces) and insinuate powerful curative suggestions to achieve intended outcomes—including outcomes like the passage of kidney stones and recovery from CNS-lymphoma. Sometimes our measures ablate noetic causes—as when we uproot a "no matter what" wish. Other times, our efforts restrict the potential for unconscious forces to find unhealthy expression—by tailoring, for example, the Principle of Parsimony to allow "Only Healthy Solutions." Always our suggestions are driven by the ineluctable law—Patterns Persist; and chief among those patterns are Authority, Linkage, and *Rapport*.

The problem with Affirmation is that once a person is rendered helpless and dependent, their own conscious affirmations are often tainted with self-doubt. Authority over oneself is diminished; susceptibility to inadvertent curses is enhanced. Regrettably, this diminution in personal power is often intensified by the Western medical establishment, which unwittingly conveys baleful warnings lest its prescriptions go unheeded. Under such conditions, while some patients may go it alone and succeed, far more will need the help of a Healer.

Remember Gene, the surgeon with warts covering his hands in Chapter 7? When I first saw Gene, his sense of agency over his health was considerably weakened. Owing to his skepticism, it took a couple of sessions and the careful cultivation of *Rapport* and Linkage before I was able to assume any real measure of Authority. Once achieved, I transferred that Authority to an affirmation infused with meaning: "warts go away…warts go away…warts go away," and so forth—10 times. In essence, that simple phrase—which you may recognize as the "Y" or consequent of our Generic Placebo Suggestion—carried with it all the curative suggestions from our hypnotic sessions. Thus, Gene was not weakly affirming "warts go away" all by himself; instead, he was echoing the words of The One least uncertain, words containing active meanings infused during trance. You may also recall this same method being used on cancer patients, with the affirmation: "Only Healthy Cells."

As a rule, I offer conscious affirmations to patients only after I have (1) applied the stamp of my Authority to those affirmations, and (2) implanted the curative suggestions attached to those words as deeply as my Authority will allow. After that, the affirmations function as the external reverberations of internalized curative suggestions.

Whenever Authority is established, this method should work. For example, the affirmations of the marvelous Louise Hay came with her imprimatur—established through the Authority vested by her readers, who knew her story and deemed her The One. The fact is, all healers command some measure of Authority, as our discussions about Placebo have established. And so, it seems reasonable to assume that the assignment of a meaning-infused affirmation by a healer stands a far greater likelihood of success than a self-generated utterance from a frightened patient with, perhaps, unconscious ambivalence.

Summing Up

In this chapter, we learned how to use the tools of the Exquisite Art to inactivate certain common noetic causes of illness and to offer generic suggestions for health and healing. The result of this approach is to restore and revivify Host Defenses. Removing frictional Zone I-Causes allows the central spin of Host Defenses to run without drag or deterioration; while adding generic health suggestions, to extend our metaphor, imparts momentum and restores Host Defenses to their natural state of vigilance and vigor.

One may argue that not all of this is needed, that we should dispense entirely with addressing discrete noetic causes and focus on commanding a cure to patients in trance. There is some substance to this argument; the work of Mesmer, Esdaile, Bernheim and countless other modern-day hypnotherapists attests to its partial validity. But why would neglecting underlying noetic causes not have the same long-term effect as neglecting underlying physical causes? A man with a rotting tooth suffers an abscess; the abscess is incised and drained. Then, because of the tooth, he suffers pneumonia; the pneumonia is treated. Then, again because of the tooth, he suffers endocarditis—a heart valve infection. At some point, it becomes clear: the infected tooth must go.

Similarly, as in Michael's case, to have ignored his guilt and other Zone 1-Causes would have been, in my view, to have invited eventual catastrophe. We will leave it to future noetic scientists to determine what can and cannot be omitted from our current method of treatment. Meantime, it is perhaps wisest for us to reprise what works—namely, discovering and addressing as many causes as possible, and treating those causes (mental and material) with whatever remedies have been proven to help and not harm.

*"You will learn more from a few failures than you will
from a thousand successes."*

—John Grinder (1985), Co-Founder Neuro-
Linguistic Programming

Chapter 13:
Limits and Failures

In Chapter I, I promised to discuss my failures and, in particular, their recurrent themes. I offer them now, with apologies to those patients I failed, and with some embarrassment before my peers. The only compensation I take is in knowing that by revealing these pitfalls, I may help others to avoid them.

Hubris (revisited)

My best case as a young Emergency Physician was, in many ways, one of my greatest failures. Worse, it was the first of several similar failures.

Doris's Story

Doris is 83 years old, and her "heart is acting up."

I introduce myself and set to work, as I had been trained—history, physical examination, laboratory tests. I discover Doris is, for the first time, in atrial fibrillation (an irregular heart rhythm). But why? There are many possible reasons—thyroid, electrolytes, heart attack, conducting system, etc.—all the blunt beginnings I had learned, and was tested on, in medical school.

Soon, her labs are back. Potassium, an electrolyte that can have profound effects on the heart, is 2.1 mEq/L—dangerously low (called, "hypokalemia"). But, as with the heart arrhythmia, why? She is on no "potassium wasting" drugs; her diet is adequate; she has no previous history of hypokalemia.

It is a busy night in the ED. I could easily admit Doris to the hospital with the diagnosis "new atrial fibrillation secondary to hypokalemia, cause unknown." This would be perfectly legitimate. But I know I have left something out, neglected one key element of the physical examination—the rectal exam. And I also know, from having read one brief paragraph in a textbook some 8–10 years ago, that a rare cause of hypokalemia can be detected by rectal examination. It is called "villous adenoma," a usually benign growth that can secrete potassium-containing fluid. Moreover, as I recall, a certain percentage of villous adenomas can be associated with cancer. I put on a glove and perform the examination.

To my surprise, something is palpable: It feels like "a wet carpet," exactly as described in the textbooks. My sense of discovery is enormous. I feel triumphant, but like many Emergency Physicians have no one to celebrate with. I finish my note and admit Doris with a five-star diagnosis: "New atrial fibrillation, secondary to hypokalemia, secondary to villous adenoma—rule out cancer."

That was the last I saw of Doris. In minutes, she was whisked to the ICU and swarmed by specialists.

Looking back, it is a somewhat shameful recollection. Though it was a busy night, patients waiting, the usual havoc—how long would it have taken to reassure Doris, before she was plunged into the maelstrom? How long to explain that her heart rhythm would most likely return to normal (potassium was being restored) and that its cause had been identified and was likely curable?

In seconds, I could have said—indeed, I should have said: "Yes, on the one hand, **some patients** with this diagnosis might have more complicated issues to deal with; but, on the other hand, the vast majority of patients—like **you**, DORIS GO ON TO LEAD A HAPPY

HEALTHY LIFE. Rest easy...I'll visit you upstairs when my shift ends."
Hope and Alliance.

I know she didn't sleep that night. I know the fear of death haunted her.

Hubris takes on many forms, but all are blind. One form, as we discussed in Chapter 3, is puffed and bloated; another, smug and self-satisfied; yet another, dismissive and peremptory. All such forms know only what they have done and pronounce it, "Grand!" None sees its imperfections or perceives the needs of its neighbors.

That night with Doris, hubris inhabited me and so filled me with self-satisfaction over a diagnosis that I was blind to the needs of an elderly woman, facing a frightful and uncertain fate alone.

Nowadays, I wrestle down the **Pride of Performance** with frequent conscious reminders that the primary diagnosis of almost every patient I see is Anxiety; and until that diagnosis is treated, the job is nowhere near complete. I also remind myself of Doris and others like her, for whom I should have done better.

Perhaps surprisingly, I also remember the baseball player Willie Mays. Remember "the catch?" (You can watch it on YouTube.) What always amazes me is not "the catch" itself, but the fact that Willie did not pause to gloat for even a nanosecond; instead, once the ball was in his glove, he whirled around and hurled it home—ever-mindful of the next play.

Willie Mays knew what all Artful Caregivers must also know—"The time to gloat is in the grave."

The Blurt

Imagine walking along a city sidewalk, somewhat unhappily, and a perfect stranger comes up to you, looks you in the eyes and says, "You are still afraid of that thing, and you needn't be." Regardless of how close to right the stranger happens to be, you will still dismiss him as insane and move quickly away. Similarly, if a friend delivers the same message at a party, it is not likely to have a deep and lasting effect—other than, perhaps, causing you to avoid that friend for a while. It is a bit like serving steak to a baby. Fed too soon, it just cannot be digested.

To have an impact, especially against deeply entrenched ideas, your ideas need to become the patient's ideas. If you have maximal Authority, you can craft your suggestions and present them directly. But if you do not, it is imperative first to cultivate *Rapport* and establish Linkage. When these steps are ignored, the consequences are at best resistance and at worst rebellion. In other words, sometimes the Exquisite Art of Caregiving requires patience.

Naturally, it depends on circumstances. Much of the Exquisite Art can be applied during the normal course of events, as outlined in Parts I and II. At such times, the moment of information delivery cannot be postponed; and so, the task of the Artful Caregiver is to meet the moment with a well-crafted and salutary message. At other times, however, it is not just a matter of "how" to craft your message, but of "when" to deliver it. In this regard, there is no better teacher than Dr. Milton Erickson. His elegant works provide abundant wisdom as to how one "builds response potential," and then delivers the message skillfully, at the optimal moment. I refer you to Dr. Erickson's rich opus for that wisdom (see Resources).

What I can teach, in this regard, is what NOT to do. Here is a classic example:

Scott's Story
Scott is a friend and colleague who has asked for help. Life isn't going quite right.

I sit with him and gather information in the manner we discussed in Chapter 8—listening for unhealthy wishes, dangerous identifications, curses, etc. Soon it is clear. Scott's "current," his parental program, is drawing him over the falls. The path his father took, the path he is on with no significant variation, is not leading him to happiness. His father was a doctor ("Dr. Smith"), Scott is an M.D. ("Dr. Smith"). His father was married, disparaged his wife and had an open affair; Scott is doing the same. The father was a perennial malcontent; Scott often despises himself and the world.

In formulating a treatment plan, I considered this: Scott is a professional. He has an advanced degree and is fairly sophisticated in psychology. And, as I said, he is a friend. I have watched him, on many occasions, draw in and utilize information with alacrity.

"So what do you think?" he asks.

I could easily have said: "Well, you know, Scott, your story reminds me of a patient…" Or, "For some reason as I was listening to you, I was reminded of these two prisoners—one who ended up being a patient of mine. Both were shackled together and kept getting in each other's way. It got so they hated each other. Only when they were finally released, which coincidentally, was on the exact same day—only then, did they realize how much they liked, even admired, each other. Not in spite of, but because of their differences." In other words, I could have offered a therapeutic metaphor. Or, building response potential, I could have said: "I'm not sure, Scott. Let me think about all this. It's really good information, and while I ponder your history, I wonder if you could spend some time asking yourself how close to completely independent do you really want to be? We'll pick this up next week.…" I could even have begun to cultivate Scott's trance-capacity, by inducing a light trance.

I could have done all or some of that, but I didn't. Instead, I convinced myself that because of his intellectual status (and friendship) he could incorporate my observations and muscle his way toward wellness independently. I knew better. I knew that regardless of one's cognitive achievements, deep change-work requires a whole different set of capabilities. Scott's very predicament spoke to his need for a powerful assist. So, why did I delude myself?

Either Scott or I, or both of us, had somehow set the expectation to "make this quick," meaning a single session. And while it does occasionally happen that only one session is required, it is not the rule. Moreover, setting that expectation is a prescription for failure. Instead of being as patient as Erickson—gently spooning therapeutic suggestions out, so to speak, as the mouth opens eagerly for another tidbit—I blurted. I detailed all the points of coincidence between his path and his father's path, and then suggested he be alert to those tendencies he disliked and "begin to blaze your own trail."

Amazed at my insight, Scott acted in every way as I might have hoped. He recited the observations, added some instances in which he now perceived the principle at work and resolved to stay alert and change the course of his life.

It was a fleeting epiphany.

Within 48 hours, the curtain of Denial descended like a guillotine— cutting off all access to his previous insights. "Oh, I remember everything we discussed. It's all about honesty," he insisted some days later, as he blindly continued to pursue his father's path.

Even "brief therapy" requires patience. It is one thing for you to know, or think you know, the causes of someone's illness. It is quite another thing for your patient to internalize and accept those ideas; and, it is seldom necessary that they do so. Erickson frequently reminded his students that a patient comes to see you wishing to move forward from place A to place B. Few people ask: "Can you take me backward, so I can review things?" (And when they do, be careful.)

Divining noetic causes can be useful in helping the Artful Caregiver to craft therapeutic suggestions, but jointly reconstructing a causal history with one's patient is a retrograde activity. Again, the patient has asked to move forward toward health. Whatever the morbid pattern, Erickson showed that constructive suggestions, not revelatory interpretations, lead most often to cure—regardless, I would add, whether you are treating psychopathy or so-called organic disease. For example, I did not say to Michael (the patient who recovered from lymphoma and graft-vs-host disease), "You are stuck with a child's view of your actions," and then leave it to him to sort things out. Instead, I first spent time gaining *Rapport* and magnifying my Authority through trance; then, using the language of the Exquisite Art, I enabled him to see and to forgive and to move past the damning events surrounding his father's demise, ultimately prescribing: *"Replacing childlike symptoms with Only Healthy Solutions...from this moment on."*

Regrettably, Scott was not the recipient of such patience. Instead, he received a few lambent insights—glancing, like light, off the surface while failing to warm the waters below.

Fortunately, I got a second chance. Months later, as his distress continued, Scott returned and I was able to perform as I should have initially. He did well, eventually setting out on his path and discovering the joyful freedom of self-determination. But second chances are rare, and I am thankful Scott allowed me the opportunity to redeem myself.

The Exquisite Art requires that knowledge of noetic causes combine with the wisdom of how and when to deliver therapeutic suggestions, to inactivate those causes. More often than not, this means patiently cultivating the moment of optimal receptivity. Then, and only then, as *Cyrano de Bergerac,* the legendary swordsman said: "thrust home."

Nowadays, I guard against "the blurt" by reminding myself that patience is truly the best expediter.

Adverse Intentions

Patients do not always approach a caregiver for help. Sometimes there are ulterior motives. The classic example is the smoker whose wife has sent him. He really does not wish to quit; but he does wish to stay married, so he agrees to "try." You know how to manage this patient and patients like him—a congruency test: Listen to his history patiently, then when you have all the usual information, thank him and say: "Now, that was all very helpful...very useful information. Thank you for being so straightforward. Please allow me to ask you just one more important question, and it's a very important question.... Are you REALLY ready to quit smoking...now?" Then, stop listening and JUST WATCH. It is as if his unconscious will speak through his head movement. If he nods, Yes, he is a patient. If he shakes, No, regardless of what he may say, you will only waste your time and his money by "trying."

Where I have gotten tripped up is not with the reluctant habit-changers; at least, not more than once or twice. But I have repeatedly blundered with patients whose problem or condition is so serious that I cannot conceive them wishing for anything but a successful outcome; and yet, that may not be their wish at all. Frequently such patients arrive in the office, not of their own volition. Instead, they come at the bidding of a familiar third party—a friend, family member or colleague, who has importuned me for their appointment. Granted, ambivalence is commonplace. But, generally speaking, if the patient has not come for help on his or her own, the balance is tilted in the wrong direction.

Here is my most recent example, the only time I have failed with pre-surgical hypnosis:

Missing the Signs

Martie is the 50-year-old wife of a physician/colleague. Her husband, a pediatrician, has asked me to see her for presurgical hypnosis, before she undergoes angioplasty of the renal artery—a somewhat delicate and risky procedure.

Theirs is a troubled relationship, characterized by much anger and frequent breakups. Martie experiencing a medical emergency is what commonly instigates their reconciliations; he alone, they both believe, can care for her properly.

Today, as in times before, he has moved out of the house, having once again declared: "I am done being your doctor."

"The hell you are," she protests, determined to draw him back—as I learned later.

Martie enters my office on time and readily volunteers her history. We agree on goals. Then, she engages in a hypnotic trance induction and appears to comply with my suggestions. There are some telltale moments, but I blindly dismiss them.

When Martie wakes, I wish her well, and it is done.

Her procedure does not go well. It is catastrophic. Martie requires several more procedures, ultimately losing the kidney, becoming drug-dependent and even threatening suicide. Her husband is with her throughout, ministering to her medical needs.

I should have known better.

These days, I do not accept patients unless they schedule their own visits. I understand ambivalence is common, but I need the desire for health to tip the balance. And so, I perform congruency checks frequently and watch closely for subtle cues of adverse intention. I wonder out loud, "Why, today?" And, I listen intently to the answer. If there are countervailing forces, they often need to be addressed first. Finally, I ignore as much as possible the pleadings of third parties.

The Limits of Physicality

Patients often present with the question, "Can your methods cure this?" If the illness is one I have treated successfully in the past, the answer is easy. If not, my approach is to recall the catalog of maladies that have been positively affected by suggestive therapeutics in order to get a sense of possibility. By now you will understand that by "suggestive therapeutics" I mean all treatments in which ideas evoke responses; this implies methods ranging from well-structured placebo-controlled trials to various imagery techniques to hypnotic trance.

Regarding Placebo Effects, the prevailing misconception is that placebo only works on psychological symptoms. For example, most doubters will concede that placebo is potentially effective against pain, anxiety, depression and other "mental conditions." But those same people are generally loath to credit placebo with improving so-called organic conditions. Of course, if they were correct, placebo-controlled trials would only be necessary when assessing the efficacy of psychiatric and analgesic drugs. In fact, we use placebo controls in virtually all clinical trials, because the evidence of the last 70 years attests to placebo's efficacy in virtually all conditions.

I grant the evidence is imperfect. For example, it would be enlightening to conduct clinical trials, wherever ethically feasible, using a three-arm approach in which one arm is the untreated disease (i.e., its "natural history," so to speak), the second arm is the test intervention and the third arm is placebo. Nevertheless, knowing that 31% of bald patients experienced "minimal hair growth" and 10% of such patients "moderate hair growth" with placebo gives us some reason to believe hypnosis might be helpful in allowing a chemotherapy patient to keep her hair throughout treatment. Likewise, a 62% reduction in the frequency of calcium oxalate kidney stones in the placebo group suggests that a properly delivered suggestion might help a patient with recurrent nephrolithiasis. And, knowing that normal saline injections in the early coronary artery thrombolysis trials actually demonstrated notable efficacy could prompt us to offer therapeutic suggestions to heart attack patients—not instead of, but in addition to conventional treatment. The point is, however imperfect, placebo-controlled trials hint at a wide range of maladies potentially amenable to suggestive therapeutics.

The hypnosis literature, which traces back centuries, can also be helpful. There is much to be learned from Mesmer and his disciples, from Bernheim and Liebault, from the great British physicians Braid, Elliotson and Esdaile, as well as from Erickson, Meares, Grinder and Bandler and all the modern healers using various forms of the Exquisite Art. Never mind their explanatory notions. Look at their results. Tumors regressed and cured; migraines, palsies, arthritides, infections, endocrine disturbances, gynecologic problems, inflammations, neurologic conditions—all remedied with therapeutic suggestions.

I also refer to my own experience. For example, I have now converted virtually every cardiac dysrhythmia, except ventricular fibrillation, using suggestion only; I have witnessed countless bloodless surgeries of the knee, shoulder and hip, as well as other major surgeries; I have seen tumors stall, regress, and disappear; seen dislocated elbow and shoulder joints reduce (i.e., relocate) spontaneously, without so much as a nudge; breech babies rotate in utero; bleeding halt; pain evaporate; wounds heal so rapidly it defies experience and explanation—all in response to suggestions. Ideas evoking responses. Most of these cases have surprised me; many have shattered my preconceived notions. As a result, I admit I do not know what limits our physicality imposes on the reach of what we today call mind. I do know those limits are far less restrictive than what I was taught in medical school—both in terms of cause and cure. And I know that this gift we call intention or will or volition—this emergent property that can influence mental and material outcomes in ourselves and others—remains incompletely explored and insufficiently explained.

All of which is to say, when a patient asks: "Can it work?" I look first at the evidence, and then if I can find none, I offer: "We are at the frontier, where miracles can happen. Shall we venture in together and discover how well it works?" More often than not, despite my barely suspended disbelief, I am pleasantly surprised.

Summing Up

Of course, I haven't listed all of my mistakes and limitations. But I have listed the ones that tend to recur, whenever I lose focus. Let's summarize:

As much as possible we need to resist **Pride of Performance,** for its momentary glare often blinds us to the urgent, unmet needs of others. As caregivers, we function best when we focus on our patients' needs—knowing there will always be time for honest self-assessment, and even a quiet bow, when the job is done.

We also need to resist **The Blurt**—remembering that patience truly is the best expediter. Understanding the cause of a malady is a bare beginning. Implementing a strategy to cure that malady is the Artful Caregiver's true task.

Finally, throughout this book we have seen how unconscious noetic factors can feature in the causal sequences leading to illness. We have discussed many of those common noetic causes—guilt, retreat into illness, dangerous identifications, unhealthful wishes. Perhaps the darkest of those unhealthful wishes is the wish to be sick or to die. As caregivers, we needn't be afraid to ask, "Do you really want to get well? Do you really want to live?" As with all congruency checks, once you have asked, stop listening. Just look. What do the nonverbal cues tell you? If the nonverbal answer is "No," that is where you must focus first.

***

Humility, patience and vigilance—cultivate these qualities along with your newly acquired communication skills and, as I wrote when we first began this journey, a universe of salutary outcomes will bloom before you and your patients.

"Above all, there will be happiness and joy of life, instead of frayed nerves, weariness and dyspepsia."

—Bertrand Russell, *In Praise of Idleness*

Afterword

We began this exploration of the Exquisite Art of Caregiving by noting that compassion is not enough—knowledge and wisdom must mingle in the mix. We found that Mind Matters; and so, avoiding inadvertent curses became our first priority. Gradually, we added the refinements of everyday communication and blueprints for waking suggestions. Our toolbox grew, and with it our ability to deliver honest information, while at the same time offering hope and alliance.

Next, we considered the Wisdom of the Body—its sacred and intricate balance. We probed the nature of symptom formation, repositioning the blunt beginnings of the reductionists within the broader context of multi-factorial causation, including both mental and material events. With these new understandings, we then examined the three phases of virtually every patient/caregiver encounter. We discovered that the entire interaction between patient and caregiver required an upgrade: Information Gathering was incomplete without asking the crucial question, "Why today?" Synthesis—the invisible process of arriving at a diagnosis, treatment plan and prognosis— required a sensitivity to the common Fallacies of Extrapolation and Prophecy, but it also required real wisdom as to the common contributory causes of illness. And when it came to Information Delivery, we learned how to say it right while standing firm and fearless in the conviction that hope for a miracle is never false hope.

Having refined our thoughts and words, we then moved on to one of the Exquisite Art's most powerful tools—hypnotic trance. Before unwinding the centuries-old misconception about hypnosis and trance, we learned why shared goals are important and why the subtleties of nonverbal communication mean we must guard against our own negative thoughts. Then, we studied trance induction and learned how to ready patients for bloodless surgeries and painless recoveries. We even plumbed the common noetic causes of recurrent illnesses and explored methods to eliminate them, and thereby produce lasting cures.

All in all, a pretty splendid path, but not without its pitfalls. I tried to point out where I had stumbled and stubbed my toes in the hope that, at the very least, you would avoid my missteps.

Only two elements remain to be discussed. The first has to do with time. The second with energy.

"The Slower You Go, the More You See"

Of course, if you are working in a busy clinic or in the Emergency Department, as I did, going too slowly can cause harm or even cost a life. The pace of practice is dictated by factors often outside our control. The key in every case is to deliver honest information with positive suggestions that leave your patients with hope and a sense of alliance. Paraphrasing Emily Dickinson: "Tell all the truth, but tell it *smart*." This requires no additional time, just the use of your toolbox—the elements of the Exquisite Art.

Going deeper, however, does require time. Time for questions and contemplation. Time to build trust and to insinuate curative suggestions. If your purpose is to discover and root out the persistent causes of someone's ill health, my experience is you will likely need at least 90 minutes for your initial visit, and between three to eight more visits of similar length to fully address the various causes. You may not become monetarily rich practicing this kind of care, but you will become wealthy. To see patients rise and walk away from the swiftly ebbing tide that nearly drew them down—that is the Healer's truest treasure. And it will be yours if you take the time to seek it.

But Not Just Time…

You will also need energy. It takes energy to interrupt your old habits and form new ones, even more energy to care deeply about others, and even more still to uncover the causes of their distress and implement cures. You cannot succeed at these tasks if you are burnt-out. For **burnout prompts exhausted caregivers to retreat behind the armored limits of the Self.**

In time, the Exquisite Art of Caregiving becomes relatively easy and habitual; however, like all complex tasks, in the beginning, it requires effort and attention. In this respect, I was extremely fortunate. Working only 12–13 shifts per month in the Emergency Department allowed me ample time for rest and study. Most caregivers are not so fortunate with their schedules. Still, I urge you to prioritize your health and happiness above all else. Take time to relax and recharge, to giggle and goof-off. Nothing is more essential to the acquisition and practice of the Exquisite Art than guarding against burnout.

Once again, compassion is not enough. The Exquisite Art of Caregiving requires knowledge and wisdom. And a crucial part of that wisdom is understanding that prioritizing your needs for rest and relaxation will ultimately redound to the benefit of all who depend on your energy and kindness.

"Life is different on the sterile end of the swab."

—Bruce Bernstein

Epilogue: For Patients

As we have learned throughout this book, a critical factor in determining a patient's susceptibility to suggestion is the degree of Authority the patient vests in their caregiver. In large part, this will flow in proportion to the degree of helplessness and dependency the patient feels. Since one day some of us may become patients, let's consider how to lessen our sense of helplessness and dependency, and thereby reduce our vulnerability to potentially adverse suggestions.

First and foremost, as a patient, it is important to realize who you are dealing with when you go to a healthcare professional. Usually, it is someone well-schooled in the treatment of certain conditions with certain preferred modalities—pills, punctures, potions, manipulations, etc. The expert will know how those conditions GENERALLY respond to their methods of treatment. That, in essence, is the core of their expertise. The expert will not know how YOU might respond to their treatment, how YOU might respond to other treatments, and often, how YOU might respond in the absence of treatment altogether.

Remember, all experts live within their skewed world of circumscribed experience, which is always biased against "spontaneous" improvements and toward outcomes predicted by the expert. The reason for this skew is twofold: First, patients who spontaneously improve do not often return to experts. Second, since the experts are often vested with Authority by their patients, their prognostications have the impact of powerful hypnotic suggestions—in essence, self-fulfilling prophecies. And since the experts have no way of distinguishing between an accurate forecast and an actualized suggestion, they naturally assume their patients' outcomes are the inevitable consequence of the way things are—the way things must always be.

So, as a patient, what can you do? The simple answer is: Do not vest Authority (as I have used the term throughout this book) in your caregivers, meaning: In matters of health and healing, do not subordinate your will to the will of others. Instead, view the individuals on your healthcare team as provisional consultants whose expertise does not include many of the immanent resources you have at your command—your "healer within," so to speak. A surgeon, for example, is retained for his or her diagnostic and technical skills. He/she offers, in most cases, very little with respect to your healing systems. You retain agency over those systems: deciding what supplements to take, what suggestions to accept or reject, what other measures might be helpful. Or, an oncologist might be required; but remember, that specialist cannot forecast YOUR outcome, know how YOUR immune system will respond, nor can he or she predict whether YOUR survival will defy his/her previous experiences. Again, to the extent possible, you retain agency over your survival systems: deciding what interventions will be performed and what will not; what internal directives YOU, yourself, will issue and what external directives YOU will accept or reject. In other words, you are not helpless and dependent. You can engage and disengage with caregivers as you choose.

Beyond that, it is fair for you to insist your caregivers NOT deliver negative suggestions. "Doctor," you might say, "in my current circumstances, I am, perhaps, more susceptible to suggestion than usual. Therefore, I need you to do everything in your power to refrain from any kind of negative suggestion or utterance. I intend to be healthy. Please partner with me and make this our shared goal." Of course, most caregivers will try their best. But even the most compassionate caregiver will occasionally misspeak. You can take this as further evidence of their humanity, of their fallibility and, perhaps, of their discomfort with uncertainty. And this awareness can further convince you that they are not infallible Authorities, but rather useful consultants.

But that is not all you can do. One of the principal teachings of this book is that Mind Matters, that conscious and unconscious ideas influence your health and healing. For example, the outcomes of presurgical hypnosis teach us that our circulatory, healing and sensory systems are all highly susceptible to the influence of ideas. Further, the myriad Placebo Effects recorded since the inception of placebo-controlled trials attest to the scope and reach of the Generic Placebo Suggestion—an idea that affects virtually every mental and physical system ever tested. Therefore, how we manage our ideas can have profound effects on our health and healing.

In this regard, I will briefly sketch out three additional measures you can initiate with relative ease to sustain health and promote healing. Of course, this is not an exhaustive list; and yet, for many, undertaking these measures will be sufficient to confer a sense of agency over your health, a sense of personal Authority—especially, as your successes accumulate, and your doubts diminish.

1. Consciously Identify and Extirpate Harmful Ideas Within You

The first measure is to consciously identify and extirpate, to the extent possible, any latent ideas within you that could be harmful. Remember, you are searching for the kind of ideas that could become contributory causes of illness. As we have learned, such ideas often assume the form of a wish: as, for example, when guilt induces the veiled wish for punishment, or when some dreaded future event engenders the quiet wish to seek refuge in the sickbed. Such wishes are often rooted in the "shoulds" and "oughts" of our early learnings; and so, sleuthing the source is often a useful step in deactivating the ideas that underlie our errant wishes. You will also want to ferret out unhealthful ideas acquired through identification: like, cigarette smoking, which is often impressed unintentionally on a child's psyche as an emblem of adulthood. Further, there may be defeatist notions that you, yourself, might have implanted during moments of disappointment or despair: notions like, "this job is going to kill me," or "this relationship will be the death of me." An honest search for unhealthful ideas, despite whatever private embarrassments may be aroused, will often drive deleterious thoughts from the shadows and into the light of consciousness.

But remember, consciousness of causes is no guarantee of a cure. Catharsis, in and of itself, is not the endpoint of this exercise, but rather, the beginning. Whatever the unhealthful ideas you uncover, they now need to be reconsidered in the context of who you have become, what you presently know and believe, who you wish to become and what your current impressions are of the sources who instilled those ideas. There is nothing magical here. In essence, this is the process of normal, healthy cognitive growth and development. You may discover that the source of an unhealthful idea was a once-revered Authority, who in your present view no longer warrants credence. Or, you may find that the unhealthful idea itself is simply untenable. Whatever the assessment, these dawning realizations (coupled with your own vigilance and determination) will allow you to initiate a process whereby previously occult impediments to health are eventually scoured away.

Of course, you may also harbor ideas that are not susceptible of conscious discovery and reconsideration. When this is suspected—as, for example, when one's medical history is a series of "endless endings," or when symptoms persist despite proper treatment—it may serve you to partner with an Artful Caregiver. Not someone who merely exhibits compassion and promotes "the Power of Positive Thinking." But rather, a person skilled in the Exquisite Art—capable of working with you to fortify Host Defenses and treat unconscious noetic causes. Of course, my hope is that eventually this capability will exist in the vast majority of caregivers. In the meantime, you will likely find an Artful Caregiver among the best of the Ericksonians and the elite ranks of those certified in NLP (see Resources). There are many others, of course, and having read this book you now have the knowledge to help you recognize them. Once you have found your Artful Caregiver, agree on your goals and pursue them together—using all of the tools we have discussed and whatever other useful assets (and there are many) your caregiver may have at his or her command.

2. Use Your Mind to Sustain Health and Trigger Healing

The second measure you can institute, after rooting out unhealthful ideas, involves using your mind to sustain health and, when needed, to trigger and accelerate healing. Such measures are variously described as accessing "the unconscious," or "the healer within," or "the innate physician." As with the first measure, this technique is from the world of "self-help" wherein many worthy methods exist (as well as numerous ineffectual approaches), but rigorous comparisons and proof of efficacy are generally lacking. While we wait for noetic science to sort out which of these methods is most appropriate for any given patient or condition, it makes sense to retain and amplify whatever techniques are already working. For example, you may have found in certain situations repetitive, unambivalent affirmations work. Initially, those affirmations might have drawn their motive force from your own personal power and/or from the influence of a revered Authority (e.g., an author, teacher, coach); and yet, with each success the technique will have acquired additional "conditioning value" through positive reinforcement. Certainly, you will want to retain and employ such useful tools.

3. Self-directed Measures

Beyond that, it makes sense to add self-directed measures that rely on proven principles. Again, there are many such techniques; and while it lies beyond our present scope to list them all, let's consider a simple Pavlovian conditioning model, whereby you associate your healthy responses to illness or injury with mental events or "thought-triggers." For example, you might choose to associate a particular word or phrase with wound healing, each and every time you suffer a cut or minor injury of some kind. In this way, you eventually acquire agency over processes that might otherwise have seemed out of reach—in essence, extending the capabilities of the "Self."

To do so, we need first to select a noetic stimulus that is (1) unique, (2) easily replicable and (3) well-timed. Why? Because, selecting a non-unique stimulus could quite possibly result in its inadvertent use, which over time would attenuate its effect. For example, if the non-unique word "heal" were the designated stimulus, then every time you think or say the word "heal," you risk inadvertently diminishing its conditioning value. Alternatively, if the nonsense word "trelnex" were selected, while certainly unique, you might easily forget it or mispronounce the word from one conditioning event to the next. That is why, as you may have noticed, I routinely suggest that patients repeat a simple noetic stimulus 10 times: "…not 9 and certainly not 11, but exactly 10 times." Thus, a common word or phrase becomes both unique and easily replicable. As to timing, the general rule is to juxtapose the stimulus in close and consistent temporal proximity to the unconditioned reflex—in this case, say, wound healing. Thus, an effective technique might be to use the word "heal" not once, but rather repeating it to oneself 10 times throughout the period during which your wound is healing. Of course, as with all such measures, the details of execution will matter greatly. But for present purposes, it is sufficient to know that such techniques can be developed with relative ease and to good effect.

Now, imagine if instead of simply uttering this noetic stimulus into the stratosphere, you direct it intently at "the unconscious"—the internal agency, charged with getting things done: "the doer," as I often call it. In this way, with each successive conditioned response (e.g., healing, recovery, etc.), that agency gains additional conditioning value. In other words, the pattern of *conscious self-direction leading to unconscious-correction* becomes established and reinforced. And, as we have learned, Patterns Persist. With proper care and cultivation, this pattern of self-directed health and healing can become one of your most precious and potent skill sets.

HEALING: BEYOND PILLS & POTIONS

Summing Up

We know the imitative propensity runs deep—that Authority and *Rapport* entrain patients to our ways. Healers who retain Authority over themselves, who admonish their own caregivers against negative suggestions, who have done the work to root out harmful ideas and trained their unconscious healing systems to respond to conscious commands—such Healers are exemplary, to both their patients and their colleagues. They are worthy of imitation. For though life may seem like a slender thread upon which we are all delicately balanced, we are not helpless in retaining that balance. In fact, there is much we can do—beyond pills and potions.

"Tell me and I forget, teach me and I may remember, involve me and I learn."

—Xun Kuang (3rd Century B.C.)

Appendix I:
Caregiver Communication Skills Testing

The following protocol is intended to assess the caregiver's skills in Information Delivery. Ideally, those skills will be taught and tested upon matriculation into a professional training school. In this way, the understandings of the Exquisite Art can provide a more humanistic context for the scientific education that will follow. For example, it would be ideal if, upon receiving their letters of acceptance, students were given *Healing: Beyond Pills & Potions* to read, study and practice. Students could then be tested on day one of their schooling. Thereafter, any deficiencies or misunderstandings could be addressed in a first-year class and retested before actual patient/caregiver encounters occur.

Perhaps one day that ideal will be met. Meantime, practitioners already engaged in patient care can use this protocol to calibrate their skills and identify their deficiencies.

I. First, No Harm
A. Your patient has a benign viral syndrome, a "cold." Inform them of their condition, your proposed treatment plan (no antibiotics) and their prognosis.

The caregiver must:

>   a. Deliver information honestly.

>   b. Demonstrate command of the distinction between "you" and "some people, some patients, others, etc."

>   c. Offer some form of placebo: an agent (supplement, tea) or activity (audiotape, nasal lavage, affirmation, etc.).

>   d. Embed a positive suggestion.

>   e. Establish a sense of Hope and Alliance.
>
>>   NOTE: Failure occurs automatically if the caregiver indulges in the Fallacy of Extrapolation or the Fallacy of Prophecy.

B. Your patient has Stage IV non-small cell lung cancer. Inform them of the diagnosis, treatment plan and prognosis.

For the sake of this exercise, assume the following:

Diagnosis—Lung cancer with metastases to the brain.

Treatment Plan—State-of-the-art, newly approved combined immuno-therapy.

Possible complications can include: death, organ damage, nausea, vomiting, diarrhea, headache and weakness.

Prognosis: The most recent large-scale study (4,900 patients) shows a five-year survival of 40%.

This scenario requires both standard Information Delivery and the informed Consent protocol, using hand gestures and verbal distinctions between "you" (the patient) and "them, some people, some patients, others, etc." Hence:

>   a. Deliver information honestly.

>   b. Demonstrate command of the distinction between "you" and

"some people, some patients, others, etc." while discussing possible risks and benefits of treatment. Employ proper hand gestures and UNDERSCORING.

c. Embed positive suggestions.

d. Establish a sense of Hope and Alliance.

> NOTE: Failure occurs automatically if the caregiver indulges in the Fallacy of Extrapolation or the Fallacy of Prophecy.

II. Refinements of Everyday Communication

A. Your patient has alcohol-induced esophagitis (i.e., "heartburn"). Offer the suggestion to refrain from drinking alcohol in three ways:

1. Directly
2. Indirectly
3. Metaphorically

The caregiver should demonstrate an understanding of these three forms of expression. He/she should also demonstrate proper UNDERSCORING in at least one instance. For example:

1. (Direct) "You know, a long time ago I gave up telling patients what they already know. Like, in your case: You have to stop drinking." (True, this is somewhat softened; but it is as close to direct as I get, unless the patient is *in extremis*.)

2. (Indirect) "I've learned that people are smart. Nobody wants things to get worse…to get an ulcer…to have a major hemorrhage. So, I've learned that people stop when YOU ARE READY. I doubt that is today. But whether it's tomorrow or the next day or the next…is a matter of personal choice."

3. (Metaphorical) "It reminds me of a little boy I knew. He didn't have a lot of money, couldn't buy but one pair of shoes per year. Interesting kid… he skipped everywhere. Didn't run, skipped. Wasn't till it was too late he

realized skipping was wearing down his heels pretty fast. At first, they were badly scuffed; but within a week or so they were ruined. Anyway, that was a tough time for him. So, he decided to GIVE UP THE HABIT, and from then on he just walked from place to place. Never saw him skip again, but he sure did smile a lot. And his shoes lasted a whole lot longer."

III. Painless Injection (volunteer subject needed)

The subject/patient knows they are about to receive an inoculation.

The caregiver must:

1. Approach the patient and introduce yourself while gaining and maintaining *Rapport*.

2. Then, instruct the patient to focus elsewhere, using CONFUSION to focus their attention: "I need you to look over there, intently, at that orange circle-square" or "Listen intently, very soon you'll hear a peculiar sound."

3. Next, the word "Just" should be used to direct and focus the patient's attention to a non-feeling modality: "Just look…" "Just listen…" "Just think."

4. Finally, as the patient becomes absorbed in that modality—i.e., looking, listening, thinking—administer a sham injection (using syringe only).

IV. The Expanded Causal Model

The scenario: Your patient has facial dermatitis, diagnosed by a dermatologist, which causes their face to appear tear-stained. The dermatologist has prescribed pills and potions, including anti-inflammatory medications and low dose topical steroids (to be used sparingly).

You have taken a history that reveals the following: The patient is working two jobs and is unhappy at both. He is staying out late, sleeping poorly and drinking immoderate amounts of alcohol. He wishes he could just quit work altogether. He feels depressed and disaffected.

HEALING: BEYOND PILLS & POTIONS

The caregiver must:

1. Draw an Expanded Causal Diagram depicting the various causal events presented by the patient.
2. Explain the Principle of Parsimony (positive and negative).
3. Discuss Ockham's razor in the context of the Expanded Causal Model.

Figure 4: Expanded Causal Model (Facial Dermatitis)

I-Causes	II-HD	III (+PP)	IV	V (-PP)	VI-HD	VII (S/S)
Exposures				All potential		"Tear" rash
Wish to Quit						Withdrawal
Retreat to Illness			Dermatitis		Weakened	
	Weakened					Depression
ETOH						
Sleep Deficit						

V. Presurgical Hypnosis (volunteer subject needed)

The subject/patient is about to undergo a simple surgery. Risks and benefits have already been discussed in detail. The patient has agreed to presurgical hypnosis as a way of potentially limiting bleeding and post-operative pain, while also accelerating recovery.

The caregiver should demonstrate an abbreviated induction. *Rapport* and Linkage should be established. Suggestions should move from description to prescription (of safe and comfortable relaxation).

The three standard suggestions (i.e., hemostasis, comfort, rapid healing) should then be delivered directly, indirectly and/or metaphorically.

Finally, whether the patient is simply relaxed or actually in a trance, the caregiver should offer suggestions to wake up. Upon the patient's awakening, the caregiver should demonstrate maintenance of *Rapport*, while saying good-bye in a manner that does not undo the work, and further, that indirectly suggests success.

Here, the caregiver must:

1. Exhibit *Rapport* building and maintenance skills.
2. Endeavor to LINK his or her words to the patient's experiences by using permissive language.
3. Move the description of present experience to prescription of future/internal experience (i.e., rest and relaxation, comfort and safety).
4. Offer indirect suggestions and, at least, one metaphorical suggestion.
5. Wake the patient and send them off, while maintaining *Rapport* and exhibiting an awareness of their suggestive power even after trance.

> NOTE: This more advanced assessment can be "optional" or reserved for the conclusion of the first-year course.

***

Once formal training of caregivers begins, the amount of information they must assimilate is prodigious. It often seems to them as if all the world's knowledge is being crammed into their heads in the shortest time possible. Much is sacrificed during those hard years of study: social interactions, sleep, laughter. Much can be lost: sympathetic capacity, thoughtful perspectives, joie de vivre. Often, one's only business is to pass today's test and move on to the next.

Many would argue, it is a necessary ordeal. But, for those who would become Artful Caregivers, there is one thing they cannot afford to lose—one thing they must not sacrifice. Student caregivers, however dehumanizing their training, must not abandon their sense of personhood to the seductive charm of material science. And so, the sooner we begin to teach them the place of Mind in the healing arts, the more likely they will be to embrace their own humanity and that of their patients.

"…we can rewrite our brains through comparatively brief, painless treatments that use imagination and perception."

—Norman Doidge, M.D., *The Brain That Changes Itself*

Appendix II:

SUGGESTIONS FOR THE ADVANCEMENT OF NOETIC MEDICINE

Throughout this book, I have worked to combine my experiences with logic and data to support the thesis that Mind Matters, that what Authorities say and do has an impact on health and wellbeing, and that healing is not just about blunt beginnings and endless endings. I hope I have given you sufficient reason to embark on your journey into the deeply gratifying and often-surprising world of the Exquisite Art of Caregiving. In a sense, since you have read this far, you now have only two options: either (1) you relapse into the habits of haphazard speech and action, knowing the deleterious effects you are likely to produce, or (2) you begin to practice the Exquisite Art with patience and humility, and marvel at the outcomes.

There is a third option, I suppose. You could dismiss it all. Accuse me, and the Artful Caregivers who came before me, of peddling poppycock. Retreat into the petri dish and from its shallows holler, "that is not science at all!" You would not be alone. But you would be mistaken.

Science begins with wonder. "I wonder what would happen if I politely command my patients to stop bleeding or to normalize their heart rhythm or to retreat into a comfortable trance?" It then proceeds to description: in this case, what are the phenomena and how were they evoked? As the descriptive phase continues, with new phenomena being described and new methods defined, attempts to explain the observations commence. Yet, as David Deutsch reminds us: "...the original sources of scientific theories are almost never good sources." This was true of Mesmer, whose "animal magnetism" theory was debunked in 1784 by the Franklin Commission. Likewise, it was true of 19th and 20th century hypnotherapists, whose conflation of trance with hypnosis—mistaking the effect for the cause—set our understanding of noetic influences back centuries. Nevertheless, now that hypnosis is understood, we can at last discern that the accounts of the ancients, the catalogs of the mesmerists, the outcomes of placebo-controlled trials—all represent a continuum of evidence attesting to the power of noetic influences on body and mind.

And so, it is time for noetic science to take the next step in its slow evolution—time for rigorous experimentation and testing. Only through controlled experiments will our concepts sharpen further and our explanations begin to attain the elegance and predictive power we consider customary of scientific theories. True, some excellent experiments with hypnosis have already been conducted; but they are few and far between. Worthy experiments on waking suggestions (i.e., non-trance hypnosis) are even rarer. Moving forward, noetic scientists will be charged first with collecting and collating whatever high quality data presently exists, and then, with proceeding to experimentation designed to support and illuminate the underlying principles of their science.

The following experiments are offered with a view to both (1) proof of principle, and (2) practicality of use. I would ask that you see these various proposals not as finished experimental designs ready for submission to institutional review boards, but rather, as rough sketches—like the first crude maps drawn by explorers of the New World—intended to impart vision and direction. As with all rigorous scientific pursuits, the devil will be in the details. And I have no doubt the details of what I am proposing will be revised and refined extensively. Nonetheless, the results of these or similar experiments will not only set noetic science on a firmer footing, they will also provide templates for future treatments to be performed by practitioners of Noetic Medicine.

Placebo: The Good, the Bad and the Usual

The notion that the placebo/nocebo response is a non-trance hypnotic response is a new and clarifying concept. It informs all caregivers of the double-edged nature of their Authority and cautions us to mind our words and deeds. The whole purpose of this book, in a nutshell, is to expose this reality and then to instruct compassionate caregivers on how to present ideas in a salutary manner that optimizes their patients' outcomes.

The following experiment is inspired by an inadvertent curse I overheard one of the best Emergency Physicians I know say to a lady who was insisting he prescribe antibiotics for her cold: "Mrs. Jackson," my colleague insisted, "as I have explained, you have a viral syndrome. Antibiotics won't help. In fact, nothing will help. You'll just have to go home and tough it out."

The Experiment

Ninety healthy volunteers receive nasal inoculations of the common cold virus. They are then randomly divided into three groups: natural history, placebo and nocebo.

Immediately following their inoculations, **Group I** (natural history) participants receive the following instructions from a white-coated Authority:

"As you know, you have all just been inoculated with the common cold virus. Because you have been assigned to the Natural History group, we will not be dispensing any medications to you. Instead, we ask that you simply record on your daily tracker whatever happens to you. Please be accurate. Thank you."

Thereafter, each day for the next 10 days these participants record their symptoms, if any, on a daily tracker.

Participants in **Group II** (placebo) receive different instructions from the same Authority:

"As you know, you have all just been inoculated with the common cold virus. Therefore, it is possible **some people** may develop some mild cold symptoms. However, you should also know that many healthy volunteers like **you** have been known to experience what is called 'subclinical infection.' That means that while they do develop antibodies to the virus, YOU DO NOT HAVE TO EXPERIENCE ANY SYMPTOMS. (sic) Others may have only the mildest symptoms for a day or two. We are giving you this placebo to take daily to help YOU STAY WELL. Please take it each time you fill out your daily tracker."

It should be noted, the first box on the daily tracker will read: I feel well. The second box will read: I have the following signs/symptoms, with a list to follow.

Participants in **Group III** (nocebo) receive yet another set of instructions from the Authority:

"As you know, you have all just been inoculated with the common cold virus. So, you are probably going to come down with a cold. We are giving you a placebo to take daily, but as you also know, viral infections just have to run their course and placebo is not real medicine, even though it can have side effects: like, headache, nausea, vomiting, etc. (list them). At any rate, you should be well again in a week or so. In the meantime, for the sake of this experiment, please fill out your daily tracker and take your placebo pill daily."

As with the other groups, Group III participants will fill out their trackers daily for the subsequent 10 days.

Now, imagine if Group III (nocebo) does worse than Group I (natural history) and Group II (placebo) does better than both. My colleague—who craves a scientific rationale but cannot logically connect the already-proven parts and pieces—will have a solid evidentiary basis for prescribing a placebo to patients with self-limited viral syndromes and delivering it with positive suggestions. So, too, will compassionate caregivers everywhere.

Informed Consent

In Chapter 5, we discussed in detail the proper way to deliver informed consent—to convey to patients both the risks and benefits of a given treatment. The refinements of words and deeds included in that protocol form the basis for much of the information delivery Artful Caregivers do in the usual course of their daily practices.

Here, I will not outline specific experimental proposals to confirm the validity of our approach. Rather, let me suggest that in order to experimentally confirm this component of Noetic Medicine, the informed consent protocol should be tested for newly prescribed medications, recommended surgeries and other common treatments and procedures. I can easily imagine such studies being conducted on antihypertensive medications, for example, where the number and degree of complications are the endpoints. Similarly, informed consent for appendectomy (or the like) would make sense—the endpoints being complications, days to the resumption of normal activities or similar objective criteria. In each case, the control group would receive the usual haphazard spew (most likely, scripted) from the Authority. The test group would receive a carefully choreographed "on the one hand... **some people** might..." presentation (as outlined in Chapter 5).

This is a relatively easy study to implement; therefore, I envision it being conducted by students in order to meet their requirements for graduation. Within a few years, we could conceivably be seeing confirmatory studies from acupuncture schools, naturopathic colleges, medical and nursing schools, and other professional caregiving institutions. This opus would, again, provide a compelling scientific basis for the practice of the Exquisite Art.

Presurgical Hypnosis

Any common surgical procedure could provide the backdrop for a clinical trial testing the efficacy of presurgical hypnosis. My experience, however, suggests that total knee replacement might provide the most salient results. Here is why. The surgery itself is often bloody; the recovery is generally uncomfortable; and return to normal activities often takes up to a year. These facts provide us with readily quantifiable outcomes amenable to comparison, especially since the most stunning results of presurgical hypnosis that I have witnessed are: (1) virtually bloodless surgery, (2) minimal requirements for post-operative analgesia, and (3) rapid recovery, including wound healing.

The Experiment

A large sample population scheduled to undergo total knee replacement (single joint) is randomly divided into two groups. The control group will see a surgeon (or another physician) the day prior to surgery and be allowed to discuss any concerns they might have regarding the imminent procedure. The test group, in addition to being permitted to ask clarifying questions, will also undergo presurgical hypnosis per the protocol outlined in Chapter 11.

The endpoints of the study will be: (1) estimated blood loss during surgery, (2) number of analgesic pills/injections used during the first post-operative month, (3) days to 90-degrees of flexion in the operated joint, and (4) days to removal of the last suture or staple.

We should understand that the two sample populations will be matched with respect to the relevant parameters, and all other necessary controls will be implemented. Outcomes on the four endpoint parameters will be analyzed for statistical significance.

Imagine if, as a result of a single one-hour presurgical session, statistically significant improvements in the study parameters are confirmed. Such results, if applied to all surgical procedures, could have an enormous economic impact on hospitals as well as the broader economy. And, for patients and Artful Caregivers, the benefits would be incalculable.

***

These are but a few of the possible experiments the concepts of the Exquisite Art lend themselves to. One can also imagine additional experiments whereby noetic stimuli ("thought-triggers") are associated with our own natural healing responses, so as to produce those responses when needed most (see Epilogue). And I am sure there are countless other studies that can and should be devised and implemented to support the principles outlined in this book. The point is, it is time—time to begin the systematic creation of an evidentiary base for the emerging discipline of Noetic Medicine.

ACKNOWLEDGMENTS

I owe an enormous debt of gratitude to my patients. They have repeatedly taught me the dangers of Hubris and the rewards of caring. Their puzzles piqued my curiosity and set me on my course. I thank them all for honoring me with their trust.

I am also immensely aware of the marvelous mentors I have had. I honestly do not know how much of this book derives from them and how much is from me. I happily share whatever credit is due for the insights and understandings herein with those magnificent teachers. However, I claim all of the errors and misstatements in this book as my own.

John Grinder taught me more in a few days about the power of ideas and their proper expression than I could have learned in several lifetimes. His many ingenious books only took it further. I thank him for his friendship and his cantankerous brilliance. Stephen Gilligan channeled Milton Erickson into me with grace and cunning. I thank Steve deeply for his lessons and skills. The Emergency Department where I worked was run by Dr. Thomas Ruben. Tom created an environment of openness and freedom that allowed me to experiment. He is gone, but I will remember him always with deep gratitude. Ron Rothenberg, M.D., journeyed into the jungle with me. Together we learned about shamanism and alternative methods of healing.

I thank Ron for his curiosity and fearlessness. My dentist, Al Mizrahi, introduced me to the possibility of painless injections. He has no idea what that led to and how many hundreds of patients have benefitted from his tenderness and patience. Rich Berlin, in my view, the greatest living doctor-poet, has been a friend of the heart since medical school. For all of us, there are times when it is hard to care and easy to retreat. Rich's indomitable love for humanity and caregiving has inspired me daily and keeps me in the game.

And how many of us are blessed with the friendship of a Taoist priest for three decades? I was. I love Sifu Share K. Lew. He was a beautiful man, and I am still learning from him. I am certain that will continue till "I go home."

Many doctor colleagues have inspired me. Chief among them is Dr. Mark Kalina. Mark taught me what is needed in medicine and, at times, what is not. If I have explained anything well in this book, it is because of Mark's influence. I have also learned from Edwin Yager, Norbert Preetz and Richard Levak—all three clinical psychologists. Thanks to you all for your lessons.

Most importantly, let me say: To have a life partner with whom to share everything is a blessing beyond words. Dianne lifts me with her enormous capacity for love and understanding. I am blessed to live in her radiance, intelligence and honesty.

To my daughters, Clea and Raquel—this book is because of you, because every parent longs for their children to live in a world of compassion, knowledge and wisdom. I hope this book will contribute its small part to the realization of that dream.

RESOURCES
RECOMMENDED READING

I. Science

General

1. Humphries, Rolfe (Translator). *Lucretius, The Way Things Are*: The De Rerum Natura of *Titus Lucretius Carus* (1968); Indiana University Press.

2. Deutsch, David. *The Beginning of Infinity* (2011); Penguin Books.

3. Kuhn, Thomas S. *The Structure of Scientific Revolutions* (1962); University of Chicago Press.

4. Feynman, Richard. *The Character of Physical Law* (1965); M.I.T. Press.

5. *NOBEL PRIZE CONVERSATIONS with Sir John Eccles, Roger Sperry, Ilya Prigogine, Brian Josephson* (1985); Saybrook Publishing Company.

6. Rovelli, Carlo. *Anaximander* (2007). Translated by Marion Lignana Rosenberg; Westholme Publishing.

7. Fleischman, Paul R. *Wonder* (2013); Distributed by Small Batch Books.

8. Durant, Will. *The Greatest Minds and Ideas of All Times* (2002); Simon & Schuster.

9. McGilchrist, Iain. *The Master and His Emissary* (2009); Yale University Press.

10. Bryson, Bill. *The Body* (2019); Doubleday.

11. Davies, Robertson. *The Merry Heart* (including: "Can a Doctor be a Humanist?") (1997); VIKING.

Causality

1. Pearl, Judea. *The Book of Why* (2018); Basic Books and imprint of Perseus Books, LLC.
2. Popper, Karl. *The Logic of Scientific Discovery* (1935); Routledge.

Conditioning

1. Pavlov, I.P. *Conditioning Reflexes* (2015); Translated by G.V. Anrep; Martino Publishing.

II. Medicine/Healing Arts

General

1. Jacobi, Jolande (Editor). *Paracelsus, Selected Writings* (1979); Princeton University Press.

2. Lamb, F. Bruce. *Rio Tigre and Beyond* (1985); North Atlantic Books.

3. Cannon, Walter Bradford. *The Wisdom of the Body* (1963); W.W. Norton Company.

4. Weil, Andrew. *Health and Healing* (1983); Houghton Mifflin Company.

5. Siegel, Bernie S. *Love, Medicine & Miracles* (1986); Harper & Row, Publishers, Inc.

6. Doidge, Norman. *The Brain That Changes Itself* (2007); Penguin Books.

7. Doidge, Norman. *The Brain's Way of Healing* (2016); Penguin Books.

Placebo

1. Edelstein E.J., Edelstein J. Asclepius: *Collection and Interpretation of the Testimonies* (1945); Johns Hopkins University Press.

2. Harner, Michael. *The Way of the Shaman* (1980); Bantam Books.

3. Program in Placebo Studies & Therapeutic Encounter (PiPS). http://programinplacebostudies.org

Body/Mind

1. Harris, Dienstfrey. *Where the Mind Meets the Body* (1991); HarperCollins Publishers, Inc.

2. Rossi, Ernest L.; Ryan, Margaret O. *Mind-Body Communication in Hypnosis* (1986); Irvington Publishers, Inc.

III. Philosophy/Literature

General

1. Russell, Bertrand. *The Will to Doubt* (1958); Philosophical Library, Inc.

2. Russell, Bertrand. *Mysticism and Logic and Other Essays* (1917); George Allen & Unwin, Ltd.

3. Russell, Bertrand. *In Praise of Idleness* (1972); Simon & Schuster.

4. Twain, Mark. *The Family Mark Twain: Corn-Pone Opinions* (1992); Barnes & Noble Books.

5. Dunn, Philip (Translator). *The Art of Peace* (2003); Tarcher/Putnam Books.

6. Rushdie, Salman. *The Enchantress of Florence* (2009); Random House, Inc.

IV. Psychology

General

1. James, William. *Principles of Psychology, Volume One* (1890); Henry Holt and Company; reprinted 1950, Dover Publications, Inc.

2. Knapp, Mark L.; Hall, Judith A.; Horgan, Terrence G. *Nonverbal Communication in Human Interaction, Eighth Edition* (2007); WADSWORTH CENGAGE Learning.

Hypnosis

1. Tinterow, Maurice M. *Foundations of Hypnosis: From Mesmer to Freud* (1970); Charles C. Thomas, Publisher.

2. Bernheim, H. *Hypnosis & Suggestion in Psychotherapy: A Treatise on the Nature and Uses of Hypnotism*, originally published as *Suggestive Therapeutics* in 1884 (1964); University Books, Inc.

3. Esdaile, James. *Mesmerism in India, and Its Practical Application in Surgery and Medicine*, published originally in 1846 (2003); University Press of the Pacific.

4. Freud, Sigmund. *The Standard Edition, Volume I* (1966). Translated and Edited by James Strachey; The Hogarth Press, Ltd.

5. Erickson, Milton H. *The Collected Papers of Milton H. Erickson, Volumes 1-4* (1980). Edited by Ernest L. Rossi; Irvington Publishers, Inc.

6. Erickson, Milton H. *Conversations with Milton H. Erickson, M.D., Volumes 1-3* (1985). Edited by Jay Haley; Triangle Press.

7. Erickson, Milton H. *Advanced Techniques of Hypnosis and Therapy* (1967). Edited by Jay Haley; Grune & Stratton, Inc.

8. Haley, Jay. *Uncommon Therapy* (1973); W.W. Norton & Company.

9. Erickson, Milton H. *My Voice Will Go with You: The Teaching Tales of Milton H. Erickson* (1982). Edited by Sidney Rosen, M.D.; W.W. Norton & Company.

The Hypnotic Method and NLP (Neuro-Linguistic Programming)

1. Bandler, Richard; Grinder, John. *Frogs into Princes* (1979); Real People Press.

2. Bandler, Richard; Grinder, John. *Trance-formations* (1981); Real People Press.

3. Bandler, Richard; Grinder, John. *The Structure of Magic, Volumes 1,2* (1975, 1976); Science and Behavior Books, Inc.

4. Bandler, Richard; Grinder, John. *Patterns of the Hypnotic Techniques of Milton H. Erickson, Volume 1* (1975); Meta Publications.

5. Grinder, John; DeLozier, Judith; Bandler, Richard. *Patterns of the Hypnotic Techniques of Milton H. Erickson, Volume 2* (1977); Meta Publications.

6. Erickson, Milton H.; Hershman, Seymour; Secter, Irving I. *The Practical Application of Medical and Dental Hypnosis* (1961); Brunner/Mazel, Inc.

7. Hartland, John. *Hartland's Medical & Dental Hypnosis* (1966). Edited by David Waxman; Bailliere Tindall.

8. Hammond, D. Corydon (Editor). *Handbook of Hypnotic Suggestions and Metaphors* (1990); W.W. Norton & Company.

9. Meares, Ainslie. *A System of Medical Hypnosis* (1961); W.B. Saunders.

The NLP Health Collaborative, a Grinder/Bostic/Carroll Enterprise

The intention of the NLP Health Collaborative is to provide the general public with access to NLP Practitioners who have received direct training from John Grinder, Carmen Bostic and Michael Carroll in the collaborative medical applications of NLP.

If you, a family member or friend have a medical condition, and you would like an NLP Health Practitioner to work with you and your physician, please visit the NLP Health Collaborative website:

www.nlphc.com

Here you will find listings of Practitioners who have been trained directly by John Grinder, Carmen Bostic St. Clair and Michael Carroll in NLP Health Applications to work with you and your physician.

Here is a short list of some simple examples of the types of collaboration among the physician, patient and NLP Practitioner:

- How to formulate questions to the physician to secure the most accurate and understandable information.
- Methods for managing potential side effects of treatments or interventions.
- The interpretation and evaluation of test results.
- Activating and optimizing complex, unconscious processes in the patient to support recovery.

Again, for these and other collaborative services, from the NLP Health Collaborative, contact: www.nlphc.com

Medical Hypnotherapists

The American Society of Clinical Hypnosis (ASCH) was founded by Milton H. Erickson, M.D. in 1957, ASCH promotes greater acceptance of hypnosis as a clinical tool with broad applications. Today, ASCH offers professional hypnosis training workshops, certification and networking opportunities that can enhance both professional and personal lives. ASCH is unique among organizations for professionals using hypnosis. Members must be licensed healthcare workers and, at a minimum, must hold a doctorate, PA Certification, APRN, CRNA or Master's degree in a healthcare discipline considered appropriate by the Society.

If you wish to find a properly trained and certified Hypnotherapist in your area, kindly go to the homepage at **www.asch.net** and click on Find a Clinician.

If you ask me my name

I will say healer, priest,

arrogant crow costumed in white,

reflecting moon.

My name is scared and distant

and sometimes too tired to care.

I am death's reluctant lover,

a child's guide, mother, father,

hero and fool. And if you like it simple,

doctor will do.

—Richard Berlin, M.D.
(Reprinted with permission)

INDEX